5:2 DIET
NUTRiBULLET RECIPE BOOK

100 Low Calorie High Protein 5:2 Diet Smoothie Recipes for Men
100 Low Calorie High Protein 5:2 Diet Smoothie Recipes for Women

RECIPROCITY

First Edition published by Reciprocity in 2014
All rights reserved

EDITOR
Phenella Atkins

WRITERS
Susan Fotherington

ILLUSTRATOR
David Joyce

Disclaimer
The information in this book is provided on the basis that neither the authors nor the editors nor the publishers shall have any responsibility for any loss or damage that results or is claimed to have resulted from reading it. Some of the recipes contain nuts or nut milk. If you have a nut allergy please avoid those particular recipes.

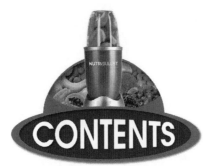

CONTENTS

All recipes are stated in Cups, Grams and Ounces.

*All recipes are stated in Cups, Grams and Ounces.
The precise nutritional break down into Protein grams, Fat grams, Carb grams, Fibre grams and Kcals is calculated for each recipe using data from the U.S. Department of Agriculture database.*

250 Kcal and 20 Protein Gram Blasts

Superfood All Round Health Boost
Made entirely out of Superfoods

Heart Care
Anti-inflammatory, high in Omega 3, anti oxidants, Vitamins C, E

Clear Thinking Brain Food
High in Omega3, Beta Carotene, Lycopene, Magnesium, Zinc, Vitamins B, C, E

Happiness, Deep Sleep and Stress Busters
High in Tryptophan, Magnesium, Vit B3, B6, B9

5:2 Diet High Protein Specials

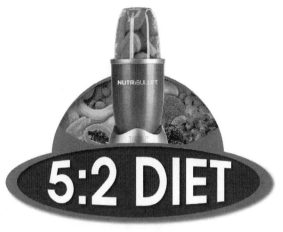

The 5:2 Intermittent Fasting Diet and Protein

It's a simple concept. You eat normally 5 days per week which means 2500 kcal with 52 grams of protein for an average 75kg/165lb man and 2000 kcal with 38 grams of protein for an average 64kg/140lb woman. Then on two days per week you restrict the calories to 25% of normal but attempt to keep the protein at 100% of normal. So you go very low calorie but normal protein 2 days per week. Men would have 600 kcal per fasting day and women would have 500 kcal. The idea behind this diet is that intermittent fasting forces the body into repair mode rather than starvation mode which is the result of continuous fasting. Therefore the 2 fasting days should be a far as possible apart from each other. Monday is not a great fasting day but the weekend is a good fasting time so perhaps Sunday and Wednesday would be good fasting days? It is your choice.

The trouble with continuous very low calorie diets is firstly that they can eat away your muscle mass which is a disaster since muscle is easy to lose but hard to regain - the 5:2 diet gets around this by doing only fasting in short 24 hour spurts, and secondly they are often deficient in protein and therefore in the 11 essential amino acids that the body cannot itself make. Our 5:2 diet NutriBullet recipes get around this by adding extra Protein (Whey, Pea, Rice or Soy). This ensures that your body gets the essential amino acids it requires on the fasting days.

The benefits of getting to the correct weight normally outweigh the dangers in successful dieting. However with a NutriBullet 5:2 diet program you are going vegetarian (or semi vegetarian) twice a week and therefore getting the advantage of raw vegetable extraction goodness on top of weight loss without protein deprivation. That should be a health bonanza!

But rather than making a tedious 100 kcal distinction between men and women Reciprocity proposes two 250 kcal NutriBullet meals per fasting day for men and for women and then men can have an extra 100 kcal of whatever they like as a bonus. Have a brunch and an evening meal. One or both of these can be NutriBullet meals, the choice is yours. However if you choose to go for full vegetarian fasting and have 2 NutriBullet 5:2 fasting meals per day, we have designed the recipes to ensure that the average person will get enough protein from these two meals.

For those of you who believe that celebrities (or their agents) have a better grasp of reality than the rest of us, the high profile 5:2 followers include Beyonce, Liv Tyler and Benedict Cumberbatch from Hollywood, the ex Scottish Nationalist leader Alex Salmond, who has lost 3 stone (and a referendum) according to the Daily Mail and the Chancellor of the Exchequer George Osbourne, who has had some success in adding the 5:2 diet program to his more general economic cut backs.

Low calorie diets are not suitable for pregnant or lactating mothers!

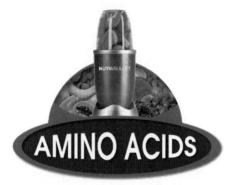

AMINO ACIDS

Essential Amino Acids

There are 11 of them: Tryptophan, Threonine, Isoleucine, Histidine Leucine, Lysine, Methionine + Cysteine, Phenylaneline + Tyrosine and Valine. These are nicely distributed throughout the leafy greens. Although meat and dairy have more protein and therefore more essential amino acids than greens per gram they have less protein than greens per kcal. So for dieters, Spinach (yummy) and Kale (fried in olive oil) are a good option.

Here are the Recommended Daily Intakes (RDI) or Recommended Daily Allowances (RDA) and Eastimated Average Requirements (EAR) for protein for 75kg/165lb men and for 64kg/140lb women.

Sex Age	EAR grams per day	RDI = RDA grams per day
165lb Men 19-30	52g	64g
165lb Men 30-50	52g	64g
165lb Men 50-70	52g	64g
165lb Men 70+	65g	81g
140lb Women 19-30	38g	48g
140lb Women 30-50	38g	48g
140lb Women 50-70	38g	48g
140lb Women 70+	48g	60g
140lb Pregnant Women	51g	64g
140lb Lactating Women	56g	70g

EAR is the estimated average requirement for 50% of people (i.e. for the average person) RDI/RDA is 20% higher and would work for 97% of the people. The figures are all linear so if you weight more then you should eat propoertionately more protein. RDI/RDA is 20% more than EAR.

The Essential Amino Acids should be eaten according to the following pattern in milligrams of essential amino acid per gram of protein intake...

Essential Amino Acid	RDI in mg per gram of Protein
Histidine	18mg
Isoleucine	25mg
Leucine	55mg
Lysine	51mg
Methionine + Cysteine	25mg
Phenylalanine + Tyrosine	47mg
Threonine	27mg
Tryptophan	7mg
Valine	32mg

So for a 75kg 50 year old man, with an RDI=RDA of 64grams of protein per day the Essential Amino Acid EARs are...

Essential Amino Acid	RDI in gram per day for a 64g perday Protein RDI
Histidine	1.15g
Isoleucine	1.64g
Leucine	3.52g
Lysine	3.26g
Methionine + Cysteine	1.60g
Phenylalanine + Tyrosine	3.01g
Threonine	1.73g
Tryptophan	0.45g
Valine	2.05g

One 200 ml glass of whole milk has between 24-42% of the Recommended Daily Intake of all of the 9 essential amino acid groups. We use 200 ml of whole milk in some of our Blast and Smoothie Recipes.

Whey protein powder (from milk) can be added to Smoothies to boost the protein content. This may be necessary for men on a low calorie diet. Good whey protein power has around 76 gram of protein per 100 grams of the powder which provides around 378 kcal of energy.

Essential Amino Acid	Grams per 50 grams of Whey Protein Powder
Histidine	0.65g
Isoleucine	2.35g
Leucine	3.95g
Lysine	3.55g
Methionine + Cysteine	1.60g
Phenylalanine + Tyrosine	2.05g
Threonine	2.5g
Tryptophan	0.50g
Valine	2.20g

50 grams of Whey Protein Powder, although having only 38 grams of protein within it will provide the full RDI of all essential amino acids for a 50 year old 75kg man except in the cases of Phenylalanine+Tyrosine where it only provides 68% (2.05g) of the RDI (3.01g) and Histidine where it only provides 56% (0.65g) of the RDI (1.15g).

This is why body builders use whey protein shakes. But low calorie dieters can benefit from them too. Women can just add 20 grams of whey protein powder and men can add 30 grams to a Nutribullet recipe and half of your essential amino acid requirements are met instantly.

Essential Vitamins

These are: A, B1 (Thiamin), B2 (Riboflavin), B3 (Niacin), B4 (Choline/Adenine) B5 (Pantotheic Acid), B6 (Pyridoxines), B7 (Biotin), B9 (Folates), B12 (Cobalamin), C, D3, E, K

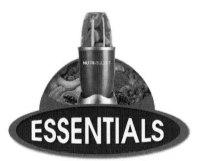

Essential Oils and Fats

This is a very short list. Basically the more fish based Omega3 (EPA DHA in particular) the better up to around 5 grams per day. And the more seed nut or vegetable based Omega3 (ALA) the better without limit.

There is plenty of evidence that Omega 3 in your diet has a large effect upon the cardio vascular system. In particular the Omega3 fish based or vegetable and seed based fatty acids should be eaten in larger amounts if you are on a high fat diet. There are good Omega3 supplements out there but whole foods containing Omega3 normally provide better absorption into the body than Omega3 supplements.

The 10 Essential Minerals

Calcium, Copper, Iron, Magnesium, Manganese, Phosphours, Potassium, Selenium, Sodium, Zinc

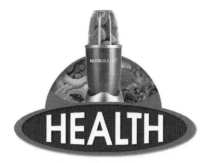

The Health Benefits of Raw Vegetable Variation

Many clinical studies have shown that raw vegetables help fight the big killers today. They help significantly to fight Cancer (the more veggies and the less meat you eat the better your body can prevent and fight tumours). There was a wonderful study done on the Norwegians during the second world war when the German occupiers commandeered all their meat. The result was that the incidence of all types of cancer in Norwegians fell by more than 50%.

They help fight Cardio Vascular Disease. They provide essential antioxidants, oils, minerals, vitamins and are generally better for us than a hamburger or a pork sausage. But the trouble is that they normally do not taste as good as a hamburger or a pork sausage unless they are roasted with cheese or boiled to the point where they have lost most of their goodness.

This is where a latest generation Blender comes in. It makes veggies taste great. A smoothie can taste as good and as invigorating as a steak with fries or a cappuccino with a croissant or a chocolate torte with cream. Your mother would never have had to tell you to: "Eat your Greens" had your family possessed a 21st century blender.

Blender manufacturers claim all sorts of health benefits from really powerful blenders. And without going into medical detail, whatever the goodness is in a vegetable or leafy green or fruit or nut or seed, the Blender can get that goodness out without destroying the delicate biochemical compounds with heat from cooking them. The modern blender has now become an extractor. This is because the machine represents the best method mankind presently has of extracting the goodness from non meat food. The blades break down the cell walls of the ingredients and thereby release the cell contents into your intestines. So unless you have teeth which can rotate at 10,000 rpm, the Blender represents a significant advance on chewing.

The other psychological trait of mankind which works against us here, is that we are loyal to what we like. Most of retail commerce is based upon brand loyalty. Although this type of loyalty doesn't always work so well with romantic partners! So we find a vegetable we like and then just eat that all the time. I mean once I have a record that I like, I will listen to it over and over again. So even if we do eat some vegetables or leafy greens or fruits, they will tend to be repetitions of a very small selection of what is available. They will just the ones that we have become familiar with and grown to like. They are essentially the vegetable next door.

So the purpose of this book is to empower to reader to vary their vegetables and fruits and greens and nuts and seeds on a daily basis. That is why we have included so many delicious Blasts and Smoothies. If you only drink a small fraction of these Smoothie recipes you will be deficient in nothing that nature provides from Vegetables, Fruits, Nuts, Seeds and Greens.

Certain amino acids (protein) and fatty acids (fat) vitamins and minerals cannot be manufactured by the body. So they have to be eaten. This is one of the reasons why food variation is so important. Failing to eat certain essential foods can be lethal – even if you are putting on weight from all the food that you are eating! This was discovered when canned liquid diets were first invented. Some of the people who tried these out continuously for more than a month just dropped dead due to running out of essential amino acids.

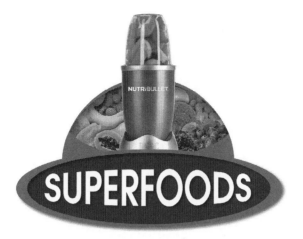

25 Widely Recognized SuperFoods

These SuperFoods contain many of the essential amino acids, fats, vitamins and minerals. But that is not why they are superfoods. They are defined as superfoods due to the health benefits that they confer. They are generally rich in anthocyanins, polyphenols, flavenoids, antioxidants, cancer fighting ellagic acid, heart disease fighting lycopene and other really useful nutrients which whilst not essential (in the sense that they can be manufactured by the body if it has the right components to hand), promote good health, fitness and well being. Between them these SuperFoods are attributed with the following health benefits…

Increased Protection from Bacterial and Viral Infections
Increased Immune Function
Reduced Cancer Risk
Protection Against Heart Disease
Slowing Aging
DNA Repair and Protection
Prevention and reduction of Cardiovascular Disease
Reduced Hypertension (High Blood Pressure)
Alzheimer's Protection
Osteoporosis Protection
Stroke Prevention
Reduced Risk of Colon Cancer
Protection Against Heart Disease
Antioxidant Protection
Prevention of Epileptic Seizures
Prevention of Alopecia (Spot Baldness)
Reduced Risk of Type II Diabetes
Reduced Frequency of Migraine Headaches
Alleviation of Premenstrual Syndrome (PMS)
Regulation of Blood Sugar and Insulin Dependence
Slowing the progression of AIDS
Protection Against Dementia

Improved Eye Health
Alleviation of Inflammation
Alleviation of the Common Cold
Improving Sleep depth and length
Detoxing and Cleasning the body
Improving Bones Teeth Nerves and Muscle

Buckwheat and **Quinoa**: Too high in carbs to be included in our list and not suitable for a Blender Recipe

Chili Peppers and Garlic: Great but not really suitable for a Blender Recipe

Almonds: High in Protein, unsaturated Fat, Vitamins B1, B2, B3, B9, E, Calcium, Copper, Iron, Magnesium Phosphorus, Potassium, Zinc and Fibre

Dark Cholcolate: High in Protein, Saturated Fat, Vitamins B1, B2, B3, B9, K, Calcium, Copper, Magnesium Manganese, Phosphorus, Potassium, Selenium, Zinc and Fibre

Flax Seeds: High in Protein, unsaturated Fat, Vitamins B1, B3, B5, B6, B9, Calcium, Copper, Iron, Magnesium, Manganese, Phosphorus, Potassium, Selenium, Zinc, Fibre

Pumpkin Seeds: High in Protein,unsaturated Fat, Vitamins B2, B3, B5, B6, B9, E, Calcium, Copper, Iron, Magnesium, Manganese, Phosphorus, Potassium, Selenium, Zinc

Chia Seeds: High in Protein, has all essential amino acids in good quantity, incredibly high in Fibre at 34%, High in Omega3 at 17%, Vitamins B1, B2, B3, B9, Calcium, Copper Manganese, Phosphorus, Selenium, Zinc

Apricots: High in Vitamins A.C, E, Iron, Potassium, Fibre

Avocados: High in unsaturated Fat, Vitamins B2, B3, B5, B6, B9, C, K Cooper, Magnesium, Manganese and Potassium, Fibre

Blueberries: High in Vitamins B9, C, K, Manganese and Fibre

Raspberries: High in Vitamins B1, B2, B3, B9, C, K, Copper, Iron, Manganese and Fibre

Blackberries: High in Vitamins B9, C, K, Manganese and Fibre

Guavas: High in Vitamins: A, B9, C, Copper, Magnesium, Manganese, Potassium, Fibre

Papaya: High in Vitamins A, B9, C, Potassium, Fiber

Goji Berries: Contains all 11 Essential amino Acids - High in Vitamins A B2 C,

Calcium, Selenium, Zinc, Iron, Potassium. But 46% Sugars. So not too many of them. Cures everything from impotence to malaria according to internet hype. Waitrose do them in the UK. Also called Wolfberries

Ginger: High in Vitamins B1, B2, B5, B6, C, Calcium, Copper, Iron, Magnesium, Manganese, Potassium, Selenium, Zinc, Fibre

Broccoli: High in Vitamins A, B1, B2, B5, B6, B9, C, K, Calcium, Iron, Magnesium, Manganese, Potassium

Carrots: High in Vitamins A, B3, B6, B9, C, K, Manganese, Potassium, Fibre

Tomatoes: High in Vitamins A, B2, B6, B9 C, Potassium, Lycopene

Beetroot: Vitamin B6, B9, C, Iron, Magnesium, Manganese, Phosphorus, Potassium, Zinc, Fibre

Kale: High in Vitamins A, B1, B2, B3, B6, B9, C, K, Calcium, Copper, Iron, Magnesium, Manganese, Potassium

Spinach: High in Vitamins A, B2, B6, B9, C, E, K, Calcium, Copper, Iron. Magnesium, Manganese, Potassium, Fibre

Swiss Chard: High in Vitamins A, C, E, K, Calcium, Copper, Iron, Magensium, Manganese, Potassium, Sodium

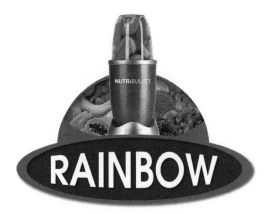

Eat a Rainbow of Colour

Red – Lyopene, anthocyanins and other phytonutrients found in red fruits and veggies. Lycopene is a powerful antioxidant that can help reduce the risk of cancer and keep the heart healthy and improve memory function.

White/Tan – Contrary to popular belief, white foods aren't so useless after all! These foods have been shown to reduce the risk of certain cancers, balance hormone levels, lower blood pressure, and boost your body's natural immunity with nutrients such as catechins and allicin. White fruits and vegetables contain a range of health-promoting phytochemicals such as allicin (found in garlic) which is known for its antiviral and antibacterial properties. Some members of the white group, such as bananas and potatoes, are also a good source of potassium.

Green – Chlorophyll-rich detoxification properties are the most noted value in leafy greens. In addition, luteins, zeaxanthin, along with indoles, help boost greens' cancer-fighting properties, encourage vision health, and help build strong bones and teeth. Green vegetables contain a range of phytochemicals including carotenoids, indoles and saponins, all of which have anti-cancer properties. Leafy greens such as spinach and broccoli are also excellent sources of folate.

Blue/Purple – Phytochemicals anthocyanin and resveratrol promote youthful skin, hair and nails. In addition, these anti-inflammatory compounds may also play a role in cancer-prevention, especially skin cancer and urinary and digestive tract health. They may also reduce the risk of cardio vascular disease.

Orange/Yellow – Foods glowing with orange and yellow are great immune-boosters and vision protectors, mainly due to their high levels of carotenoids. Carotenoids give this group their vibrant colour. A well-known carotenoid called Betacarotene is found in sweet potatoes, pumpkins and carrots. It is converted to vitamin A, which helps maintain healthy mucous membranes and healthy eyes. Another carotenoid called lutein is stored in the eye and has been found to prevent cataracts and age-related macular degeneration, which can lead to blindness.

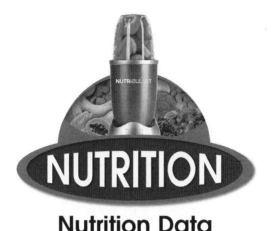

Nutrition Data

All our Blasts and Smoothies come with full nutritional data giving the precise number of grams of Protein, Carbohydrate, Fat and Fibre for each recipe and the number of Kcals it contains. The data is taken mainly from the USDA database.

Warnings

Do not put your hand or any implement near the blades when the Blender is plugged in to an electricity supply.

Authors Preference for Kale

Kale is a Superfood and is very good for you. But it does not taste as good as the other greens in a Smoothie in our opinion! To be frank, it tastes like cardboard. So we have excluded it from these recipes. It is better to fry it in some olive oil.

AVOID THESE INGREDIENTS: Apple Pear Peach Plum Apricot and Cherry **stones and pips** contain cyanide which is very poisonous. These stones and pips *must* therefore be removed before use!

Rhubarb leaves contain oxalate which causes kidney stones, comas, convulsions. 5lb of Rhubarb leaves is fatal!

Tomatoes are fine but the **tomato leaves and vines** are not. They contain alkaloid poisons such as atropine which causes headaches dizziness and vomiting.

Nutmeg: Contains myristicine which is halucingoenic and causes dizziness and vomiting. It is OK in small quantities as a spice but we do not recommend it for a Smoothie.

Kidney Beans and **Lima Beans**: These are really really poisonous if eaten raw.

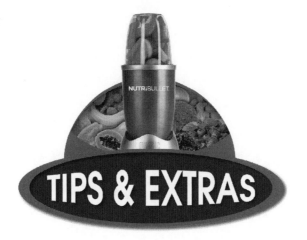

Tips and Extras

Cinnamon and Cloves are lovely in a hot drink but do not really work in a cold one such as a Smoothie. We cannot recommend adding sugar given the health difficulties associated with refined sucrose. But the following are fantastic in Smoothies...

Ginger Root (sliced up)
Lemon Juice
Lime Juice
Agave Nectar
Honey
Garlic Cloves
Cocoa Powder which is also called Cacao Powder (a Superfood)
85% Dark Chocolate (a Superfood)
Instant Coffee
Coriander
Parsley
Sage
Chives
Whey Protein (Banana, Chocolate, Cookies, Strawberry flavours etc.) – for extra protein

These can be added to any of the recipes for taste.

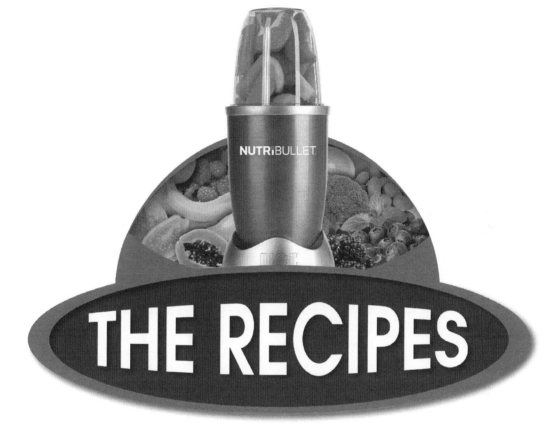

Superfood All Round Health Boost *Made entirely out of Superfoods*

Apricot Treat

Ingredients

1 Cup/Handful of Swiss Chard (40 grams or 1½ oz)
1 Cup/Handful of Spinach (40 grams or 1½ oz)
1½ Cups of Apricot halves (180 grams or 6 oz)
200 ml / 7 fl oz of Water
25 grams or ¾ oz of Pea Protein
8 grams or 0.28 oz of Pumpkin Seeds

Protein 26g, Fat 5g, Carb 21g, Fibre 6g, 250 Kcals

Preparation

Place the nuts or seeds into the Tall Cup. Screw the Nutribullet Extractor Blade on to the top of the cup. Invert the cup, press it down into the Nutribullet Power Base and twist it into place. Blast them for 30 seconds. Put the rest of the solid ingredients into the cup and press them down below the Max Line. Add the fluid base to fill the cup up to the Max Line. Screw the Nutribullet Extractor Blade on to the top of the cup. Invert the cup, press it down into the Nutribullet Power Base and twist it into place. Blast the mixture until it is really smooth (20 or so seconds). ***Enjoy!***

Blueberry Utopia

Ingredients

1 Cup/Handful of Broccoli Florets (40 grams or 1½ oz)
1 Cup/Handful of Spinach (40 grams or 1½ oz)
¾ Cup of Blueberries (90 grams or 3 oz)
¾ Cup of Blackberries (90 grams or 3 oz)
200 ml / 7 fl oz of Almond Milk (Unsweetened)
22 grams or ¾ oz of Soy Protein
5 grams or 0.18 oz of Flax Seeds

Protein 26g, Fat 5g, Carb 18g, Fibre 11g, 250 Kcals

Preparation

Place the nuts or seeds into the Tall Cup. Screw the Nutribullet Extractor Blade on to the top of the cup. Invert the cup, press it down into the Nutribullet Power Base and twist it into place. Blast them for 30 seconds. Put the rest of the solid ingredients into the cup and press them down below the Max Line. Add the fluid base to fill the cup up to the Max Line. Screw the Nutribullet Extractor Blade on to the top of the cup. Invert the cup, press it down into the Nutribullet Power Base and twist it into place. Blast the mixture until it is really smooth (20 or so seconds). ***Enjoy!***

Chard Sunrise

Ingredients

1 Cup/Handful of Swiss Chard (40 grams or 1½ oz)
1 Cup/Handful of Broccoli Florets (40 grams or 1½ oz)
1½ Cups of Guava (180 grams or 6 oz)
200 ml / 7 fl oz of Water
25 grams or ¾ oz of Pea Protein
1 gram or 0.04 oz of Pumpkin Seeds

Protein 26g, Fat 3g, Carb 21g, Fibre 11g, 251 Kcals

Preparation

Place the nuts or seeds into the Tall Cup. Screw the Nutribullet Extractor Blade on to the top of the cup. Invert the cup, press it down into the Nutribullet Power Base and twist it into place. Blast them for 30 seconds. Put the rest of the solid ingredients into the cup and press them down below the Max Line. Add the fluid base to fill the cup up to the Max Line. Screw the Nutribullet Extractor Blade on to the top of the cup. Invert the cup, press it down into the Nutribullet Power Base and twist it into place. Blast the mixture until it is really smooth (20 or so seconds). **Enjoy!**

Chard and Broccoli Vortex

Ingredients

1 Cup/Handful of Swiss Chard (40 grams or 1½ oz)
1 Cup/Handful of Broccoli Florets (40 grams or 1½ oz)
¾ Cup of Blueberries (90 grams or 3 oz)
¾ Cup of Apricot halves (90 grams or 3 oz)
200 ml / 7 fl oz of Water
22 grams or ¾ oz of Soy Protein
9 grams or 0.32 oz of Pumpkin Seeds

Protein 26g, Fat 5g, Carb 24g, Fibre 6g, 251 Kcals

Preparation

Place the nuts or seeds into the Tall Cup. Screw the Nutribullet Extractor Blade on to the top of the cup. Invert the cup, press it down into the Nutribullet Power Base and twist it into place. Blast them for 30 seconds. Put the rest of the solid ingredients into the cup and press them down below the Max Line. Add the fluid base to fill the cup up to the Max Line. Screw the Nutribullet Extractor Blade on to the top of the cup. Invert the cup, press it down into the Nutribullet Power Base and twist it into place. Blast the mixture until it is really smooth (20 or so seconds). **Enjoy!**

Broccoli Sonata

Ingredients

1 Cup/Handful of Broccoli Florets (40 grams or 1½ oz)
1 Cup/Handful of Spinach (40 grams or 1½ oz)
¾ Cup of Raspberries (90 grams or 3 oz)
¾ Cup of Blackberries (90 grams or 3 oz)
200 ml / 7 fl oz of Almond Milk (Unsweetened)
25 grams or ¾ oz of Rice Protein
5 grams or 0.18 oz of Chia Seeds

Protein 26g, Fat 5g, Carb 14g, Fibre 15g, 251 Kcals

Preparation

Place the nuts or seeds into the Tall Cup. Screw the Nutribullet Extractor Blade on to the top of the cup. Invert the cup, press it down into the Nutribullet Power Base and twist it into place. Blast them for 30 seconds. Put the rest of the solid ingredients into the cup and press them down below the Max Line. Add the fluid base to fill the cup up to the Max Line. Screw the Nutribullet Extractor Blade on to the top of the cup. Invert the cup, press it down into the Nutribullet Power Base and twist it into place. Blast the mixture until it is really smooth (20 or so seconds). **Enjoy!**

Blackberry and Papaya Fandango

Ingredients

1 Cup/Handful of Broccoli Florets (40 grams or 1½ oz)
1 Cup/Handful of Swiss Chard (40 grams or 1½ oz)
¾ Cup of Blackberries (90 grams or 3 oz)
¾ Cup of Papaya (90 grams or 3 oz)
200 ml / 7 fl oz of Water
22 grams or ¾ oz of Soy Protein
13 grams or 0.46 oz of Flax Seeds

Protein 26g, Fat 6g, Carb 16g, Fibre 12g, 253 Kcals

Preparation

Place the nuts or seeds into the Tall Cup. Screw the Nutribullet Extractor Blade on to the top of the cup. Invert the cup, press it down into the Nutribullet Power Base and twist it into place. Blast them for 30 seconds. Put the rest of the solid ingredients into the cup and press them down below the Max Line. Add the fluid base to fill the cup up to the Max Line. Screw the Nutribullet Extractor Blade on to the top of the cup. Invert the cup, press it down into the Nutribullet Power Base and twist it into place. Blast the mixture until it is really smooth (20 or so seconds). **Enjoy!**

Papaya Seduction

Ingredients

1 Cup/Handful of Broccoli Florets (40 grams or 1½ oz)
1 Cup/Handful of Swiss Chard (40 grams or 1½ oz)
¾ Cup of Raspberries (90 grams or 3 oz)
¾ Cup of Papaya (90 grams or 3 oz)
200 ml / 7 fl oz of Almond Milk (Unsweetened)
25 grams or ¾ oz of Whey Protein
5 grams or 0.18 oz of Flax Seeds

Protein 24g, Fat 7g, Carb 18g, Fibre 13g, 253 Kcals

Preparation

Place the nuts or seeds into the Tall Cup. Screw the Nutribullet Extractor Blade on to the top of the cup. Invert the cup, press it down into the Nutribullet Power Base and twist it into place. Blast them for 30 seconds. Put the rest of the solid ingredients into the cup and press them down below the Max Line. Add the fluid base to fill the cup up to the Max Line. Screw the Nutribullet Extractor Blade on to the top of the cup. Invert the cup, press it down into the Nutribullet Power Base and twist it into place. Blast the mixture until it is really smooth (20 or so seconds). **Enjoy!**

Blackberry Elixir

Ingredients

1 Cup/Handful of Broccoli Florets (40 grams or 1½ oz)
1 Cup/Handful of Swiss Chard (40 grams or 1½ oz)
¾ Cup of Blueberries (90 grams or 3 oz)
¾ Cup of Blackberries (90 grams or 3 oz)
200 ml / 7 fl oz of Water
25 grams or ¾ oz of Pea Protein
7 grams or 0.25 oz of Almonds

Protein 25g, Fat 5g, Carb 20g, Fibre 9g, 254 Kcals

Preparation

Place the nuts or seeds into the Tall Cup. Screw the Nutribullet Extractor Blade on to the top of the cup. Invert the cup, press it down into the Nutribullet Power Base and twist it into place. Blast them for 30 seconds. Put the rest of the solid ingredients into the cup and press them down below the Max Line. Add the fluid base to fill the cup up to the Max Line. Screw the Nutribullet Extractor Blade on to the top of the cup. Invert the cup, press it down into the Nutribullet Power Base and twist it into place. Blast the mixture until it is really smooth (20 or so seconds). **Enjoy!**

Spinach Mirage

Ingredients

1 Cup/Handful of Spinach (40 grams or 1½ oz)
1 Cup/Handful of Broccoli Florets (40 grams or 1½ oz)
¾ Cup of Apricot halves (90 grams or 3 oz)
¾ Cup of Blueberries (90 grams or 3 oz)
200 ml / 7 fl oz of Almond Milk (Unsweetened)
25 grams or ¾ oz of Pea Protein
2 grams or 0.07 oz of Chia Seeds

Protein 25g, Fat 5g, Carb 24g, Fibre 7g, 254 Kcals

Preparation

Place the nuts or seeds into the Tall Cup. Screw the Nutribullet Extractor Blade on to the top of the cup. Invert the cup, press it down into the Nutribullet Power Base and twist it into place. Blast them for 30 seconds. Put the rest of the solid ingredients into the cup and press them down below the Max Line. Add the fluid base to fill the cup up to the Max Line. Screw the Nutribullet Extractor Blade on to the top of the cup. Invert the cup, press it down into the Nutribullet Power Base and twist it into place. Blast the mixture until it is really smooth (20 or so seconds). *Enjoy!*

Guava Blend

Ingredients

1 Cup/Handful of Broccoli Florets (40 grams or 1½ oz)
1 Cup/Handful of Spinach (40 grams or 1½ oz)
¾ Cup of Guava (90 grams or 3 oz)
¾ Cup of Blackberries (90 grams or 3 oz)
200 ml / 7 fl oz of Almond Milk (Unsweetened)
25 grams or ¾ oz of Whey Protein
2 grams or 0.07 oz of Almonds

Protein 26g, Fat 6g, Carb 16g, Fibre 14g, 255 Kcals

Preparation

Place the nuts or seeds into the Tall Cup. Screw the Nutribullet Extractor Blade on to the top of the cup. Invert the cup, press it down into the Nutribullet Power Base and twist it into place. Blast them for 30 seconds. Put the rest of the solid ingredients into the cup and press them down below the Max Line. Add the fluid base to fill the cup up to the Max Line. Screw the Nutribullet Extractor Blade on to the top of the cup. Invert the cup, press it down into the Nutribullet Power Base and twist it into place. Blast the mixture until it is really smooth (20 or so seconds). *Enjoy!*

Guava kisses Tomato

Ingredients

2 Cups/Handfuls of Broccoli Florets (80 grams or 3 oz)
¾ Cup of Guava (90 grams or 3 oz)
¾ Cup of sliced Tomato (90 grams or 3 oz)
200 ml / 7 fl oz of Almond Milk (Unsweetened)
25 grams or ¾ oz of Pea Protein
3 grams or 0.11 oz of Almonds

Protein 26g, Fat 6g, Carb 17g, Fibre 9g, 250 Kcals

Preparation

Place the nuts or seeds into the Tall Cup. Screw the Nutribullet Extractor Blade on to the top of the cup. Invert the cup, press it down into the Nutribullet Power Base and twist it into place. Blast them for 30 seconds. Put the rest of the solid ingredients into the cup and press them down below the Max Line. Add the fluid base to fill the cup up to the Max Line. Screw the Nutribullet Extractor Blade on to the top of the cup. Invert the cup, press it down into the Nutribullet Power Base and twist it into place. Blast the mixture until it is really smooth (20 or so seconds). **Enjoy!**

Chard and Broccoli Revelation

Ingredients

1 Cup/Handful of Swiss Chard (40 grams or 1½ oz)
1 Cup/Handful of Broccoli Florets (40 grams or 1½ oz)
¾ Cup of Blackberries (90 grams or 3 oz)
¾ Cup of sliced Tomato (90 grams or 3 oz)
200 ml / 7 fl oz of Almond Milk (Unsweetened)
25 grams or ¾ oz of Whey Protein
11 grams or 0.39 oz of Chia Seeds

Protein 26g, Fat 8g, Carb 12g, Fibre 14g, 250 Kcals

Preparation

Place the nuts or seeds into the Tall Cup. Screw the Nutribullet Extractor Blade on to the top of the cup. Invert the cup, press it down into the Nutribullet Power Base and twist it into place. Blast them for 30 seconds. Put the rest of the solid ingredients into the cup and press them down below the Max Line. Add the fluid base to fill the cup up to the Max Line. Screw the Nutribullet Extractor Blade on to the top of the cup. Invert the cup, press it down into the Nutribullet Power Base and twist it into place. Blast the mixture until it is really smooth (20 or so seconds). **Enjoy!**

Carrot Tonic

Ingredients

1 Cup/Handful of Swiss Chard (40 grams or 1½ oz)
1 Cup/Handful of Broccoli Florets (40 grams or 1½ oz)
¾ Cup of Raspberries (90 grams or 3 oz)
¾ Cup of sliced Carrots (90 grams or 3 oz)
200 ml / 7 fl oz of Water
25 grams or ¾ oz of Whey Protein
9 grams or 0.32 oz of Pumpkin Seeds

Protein 25g, Fat 6g, Carb 16g, Fibre 12g, 250 Kcals

Preparation

Place the nuts or seeds into the Tall Cup. Screw the Nutribullet Extractor Blade on to the top of the cup. Invert the cup, press it down into the Nutribullet Power Base and twist it into place. Blast them for 30 seconds. Put the rest of the solid ingredients into the cup and press them down below the Max Line. Add the fluid base to fill the cup up to the Max Line. Screw the Nutribullet Extractor Blade on to the top of the cup. Invert the cup, press it down into the Nutribullet Power Base and twist it into place. Blast the mixture until it is really smooth (20 or so seconds). **Enjoy!**

Broccoli and Guava Concerto

Ingredients

1 Cup/Handful of Spinach (40 grams or 1½ oz)
1 Cup/Handful of Broccoli Florets (40 grams or 1½ oz)
¾ Cup of Guava (90 grams or 3 oz)
¾ Cup of sliced Carrots (90 grams or 3 oz)
200 ml / 7 fl oz of Almond Milk (Unsweetened)
25 grams or ¾ oz of Rice Protein
2 grams or 0.07 oz of Almonds

Protein 27g, Fat 5g, Carb 19g, Fibre 10g, 251 Kcals

Preparation

Place the nuts or seeds into the Tall Cup. Screw the Nutribullet Extractor Blade on to the top of the cup. Invert the cup, press it down into the Nutribullet Power Base and twist it into place. Blast them for 30 seconds. Put the rest of the solid ingredients into the cup and press them down below the Max Line. Add the fluid base to fill the cup up to the Max Line. Screw the Nutribullet Extractor Blade on to the top of the cup. Invert the cup, press it down into the Nutribullet Power Base and twist it into place. Blast the mixture until it is really smooth (20 or so seconds). **Enjoy!**

Apricot Wonder

Ingredients

1 Cup/Handful of Broccoli Florets (40 grams or 1½ oz)
1 Cup/Handful of Spinach (40 grams or 1½ oz)
¾ Cup of Apricot halves (90 grams or 3 oz)
¾ Cup of sliced Carrots (90 grams or 3 oz)
200 ml / 7 fl oz of Almond Milk (Unsweetened)
25 grams or ¾ oz of Whey Protein
6 grams or 0.21 oz of Chia Seeds

Protein 25g, Fat 6g, Carb 19g, Fibre 11g, 252 Kcals

Preparation

Place the nuts or seeds into the Tall Cup. Screw the Nutribullet Extractor Blade on to the top of the cup. Invert the cup, press it down into the Nutribullet Power Base and twist it into place. Blast them for 30 seconds. Put the rest of the solid ingredients into the cup and press them down below the Max Line. Add the fluid base to fill the cup up to the Max Line. Screw the Nutribullet Extractor Blade on to the top of the cup. Invert the cup, press it down into the Nutribullet Power Base and twist it into place. Blast the mixture until it is really smooth (20 or so seconds). **Enjoy!**

Raspberry and Carrot Forever

Ingredients

2 Cups/Handfuls of Broccoli Florets (80 grams or 3 oz)
¾ Cup of Raspberries (90 grams or 3 oz)
¾ Cup of sliced Carrots (90 grams or 3 oz)
200 ml / 7 fl oz of Almond Milk (Unsweetened)
25 grams or ¾ oz of Whey Protein
4 grams or 0.14 oz of Flax Seeds

Protein 25g, Fat 6g, Carb 16g, Fibre 14g, 252 Kcals

Preparation

Place the nuts or seeds into the Tall Cup. Screw the Nutribullet Extractor Blade on to the top of the cup. Invert the cup, press it down into the Nutribullet Power Base and twist it into place. Blast them for 30 seconds. Put the rest of the solid ingredients into the cup and press them down below the Max Line. Add the fluid base to fill the cup up to the Max Line. Screw the Nutribullet Extractor Blade on to the top of the cup. Invert the cup, press it down into the Nutribullet Power Base and twist it into place. Blast the mixture until it is really smooth (20 or so seconds). **Enjoy!**

Spinach and Papaya Contradiction

Ingredients

1 Cup/Handful of Broccoli Florets (40 grams or 1½ oz)
1 Cup/Handful of Spinach (40 grams or 1½ oz)
¾ Cup of Papaya (90 grams or 3 oz)
¾ Cup of diced Beetroot (90 grams or 3 oz)
200 ml / 7 fl oz of Water
25 grams or ¾ oz of Pea Protein
9 grams or 0.32 oz of Pumpkin Seeds

Protein 26g, Fat 5g, Carb 20g, Fibre 6g, 252 Kcals

Preparation

Place the nuts or seeds into the Tall Cup. Screw the Nutribullet Extractor Blade on to the top of the cup. Invert the cup, press it down into the Nutribullet Power Base and twist it into place. Blast them for 30 seconds. Put the rest of the solid ingredients into the cup and press them down below the Max Line. Add the fluid base to fill the cup up to the Max Line. Screw the Nutribullet Extractor Blade on to the top of the cup. Invert the cup, press it down into the Nutribullet Power Base and twist it into place. Blast the mixture until it is really smooth (20 or so seconds). ***Enjoy!***

Spinach hugs Apricot

Ingredients

1 Cup/Handful of Broccoli Florets (40 grams or 1½ oz)
1 Cup/Handful of Spinach (40 grams or 1½ oz)
¾ Cup of Apricot halves (90 grams or 3 oz)
¾ Cup of diced Beetroot (90 grams or 3 oz)
200 ml / 7 fl oz of Almond Milk (Unsweetened)
25 grams or ¾ oz of Rice Protein
6 grams or 0.21 oz of Chia Seeds

Protein 27g, Fat 5g, Carb 20g, Fibre 9g, 253 Kcals

Preparation

Place the nuts or seeds into the Tall Cup. Screw the Nutribullet Extractor Blade on to the top of the cup. Invert the cup, press it down into the Nutribullet Power Base and twist it into place. Blast them for 30 seconds. Put the rest of the solid ingredients into the cup and press them down below the Max Line. Add the fluid base to fill the cup up to the Max Line. Screw the Nutribullet Extractor Blade on to the top of the cup. Invert the cup, press it down into the Nutribullet Power Base and twist it into place. Blast the mixture until it is really smooth (20 or so seconds). ***Enjoy!***

Blackberry and Beetroot Treat

Ingredients

2 Cups/Handfuls of Spinach (80 grams or 3 oz)
¾ Cup of Blackberries (90 grams or 3 oz)
¾ Cup of diced Beetroot (90 grams or 3 oz)
200 ml / 7 fl oz of Water
25 grams or ¾ oz of Rice Protein
12 grams or 0.42 oz of Flax Seeds

Protein 27g, Fat 6g, Carb 14g, Fibre 12g, 253 Kcals

Preparation

Place the nuts or seeds into the Tall Cup. Screw the Nutribullet Extractor Blade on to the top of the cup. Invert the cup, press it down into the Nutribullet Power Base and twist it into place. Blast them for 30 seconds. Put the rest of the solid ingredients into the cup and press them down below the Max Line. Add the fluid base to fill the cup up to the Max Line. Screw the Nutribullet Extractor Blade on to the top of the cup. Invert the cup, press it down into the Nutribullet Power Base and twist it into place. Blast the mixture until it is really smooth (20 or so seconds). **Enjoy!**

Spinach meets Blueberry

Ingredients

1 Cup/Handful of Spinach (40 grams or 1½ oz)
1 Cup/Handful of Swiss Chard (40 grams or 1½ oz)
¾ Cup of Blueberries (90 grams or 3 oz)
¾ Cup of diced Beetroot (90 grams or 3 oz)
200 ml / 7 fl oz of Water
22 grams or ¾ oz of Soy Protein
11 grams or 0.39 oz of Pumpkin Seeds

Protein 26g, Fat 6g, Carb 21g, Fibre 7g, 254 Kcals

Preparation

Place the nuts or seeds into the Tall Cup. Screw the Nutribullet Extractor Blade on to the top of the cup. Invert the cup, press it down into the Nutribullet Power Base and twist it into place. Blast them for 30 seconds. Put the rest of the solid ingredients into the cup and press them down below the Max Line. Add the fluid base to fill the cup up to the Max Line. Screw the Nutribullet Extractor Blade on to the top of the cup. Invert the cup, press it down into the Nutribullet Power Base and twist it into place. Blast the mixture until it is really smooth (20 or so seconds). **Enjoy!**

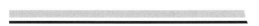

Heart Care
Anti-inflammatory, high in Omega 3, anti oxidants, Vitamins C, E

Tangerine and Carrot Delight

Ingredients

2 Cups/Handfuls of Spinach (80 grams or 3 oz)
¾ Cup of Tangerine slices (90 grams or 3 oz)
¾ Cup of sliced Carrots (90 grams or 3 oz)
200 ml / 7 fl oz of Almond Milk (Unsweetened)
22 grams or ¾ oz of Soy Protein
6 grams or 0.21 oz of Sesame Seeds Hulled

Protein 26g, Fat 7g, Carb 19g, Fibre 7g, 250 Kcals

Preparation

Place the nuts or seeds into the Tall Cup. Screw the Nutribullet Extractor Blade on to the top of the cup. Invert the cup, press it down into the Nutribullet Power Base and twist it into place. Blast them for 30 seconds. Put the rest of the solid ingredients into the cup and press them down below the Max Line. Add the fluid base to fill the cup up to the Max Line. Screw the Nutribullet Extractor Blade on to the top of the cup. Invert the cup, press it down into the Nutribullet Power Base and twist it into place. Blast the mixture until it is really smooth (20 or so seconds). **Enjoy!**

Lettuce and Tangerine Sunset

Ingredients

1 Cup/Handful of Spinach (40 grams or 1½ oz)
1 Cup/Handful of Lettuce Leaves (40 grams or 1½ oz)
¾ Cup of Tangerine slices (90 grams or 3 oz)
¾ Cup of sliced Carrots (90 grams or 3 oz)
200 ml / 7 fl oz of Almond Milk (Unsweetened)
25 grams or ¾ oz of Whey Protein
6 grams or 0.21 oz of Chia Seeds

Protein 24g, Fat 6g, Carb 20g, Fibre 11g, 250 Kcals

Preparation

Place the nuts or seeds into the Tall Cup. Screw the Nutribullet Extractor Blade on to the top of the cup. Invert the cup, press it down into the Nutribullet Power Base and twist it into place. Blast them for 30 seconds. Put the rest of the solid ingredients into the cup and press them down below the Max Line. Add the fluid base to fill the cup up to the Max Line. Screw the Nutribullet Extractor Blade on to the top of the cup. Invert the cup, press it down into the Nutribullet Power Base and twist it into place. Blast the mixture until it is really smooth (20 or so seconds). **Enjoy!**

Strawberry and Carrot Salad

Ingredients

2 Cups/Handfuls of Rocket/Arugura Lettuce (80 grams or 3 oz)
¾ Cup of Strawberries (90 grams or 3 oz)
¾ Cup of sliced Carrots (90 grams or 3 oz)
200 ml / 7 fl oz of Almond Milk (Unsweetened)
25 grams or ¾ oz of Whey Protein
11 grams or 0.39 oz of Chia Seeds

Protein 24g, Fat 7g, Carb 15g, Fibre 12g, 251 Kcals

Preparation

Place the nuts or seeds into the Tall Cup. Screw the Nutribullet Extractor Blade on to the top of the cup. Invert the cup, press it down into the Nutribullet Power Base and twist it into place. Blast them for 30 seconds. Put the rest of the solid ingredients into the cup and press them down below the Max Line. Add the fluid base to fill the cup up to the Max Line. Screw the Nutribullet Extractor Blade on to the top of the cup. Invert the cup, press it down into the Nutribullet Power Base and twist it into place. Blast the mixture until it is really smooth (20 or so seconds). **Enjoy!**

Rocket Ensemble

Ingredients

1 Cup/Handful of Broccoli Florets (40 grams or 1½ oz)
1 Cup/Handful of Rocket/Arugura Lettuce (40 grams or 1½ oz)
¾ Cup of Strawberries (90 grams or 3 oz)
¾ Cup of sliced Carrots (90 grams or 3 oz)
200 ml / 7 fl oz of Almond Milk (Unsweetened)
25 grams or ¾ oz of Rice Protein
9 grams or 0.32 oz of Flax Seeds

Protein 26g, Fat 7g, Carb 16g, Fibre 9g, 252 Kcals

Preparation

Place the nuts or seeds into the Tall Cup. Screw the Nutribullet Extractor Blade on to the top of the cup. Invert the cup, press it down into the Nutribullet Power Base and twist it into place. Blast them for 30 seconds. Put the rest of the solid ingredients into the cup and press them down below the Max Line. Add the fluid base to fill the cup up to the Max Line. Screw the Nutribullet Extractor Blade on to the top of the cup. Invert the cup, press it down into the Nutribullet Power Base and twist it into place. Blast the mixture until it is really smooth (20 or so seconds). **Enjoy!**

Spinach Forever

Ingredients

1 Cup/Handful of Spinach (40 grams or 1½ oz)
1 Cup/Handful of Lettuce Leaves (40 grams or 1½ oz)
¾ Cup of Guava (90 grams or 3 oz)
¾ Cup of sliced Cauliflower florets (90 grams or 3 oz)
200 ml / 7 fl oz of Almond Milk (Unsweetened)
25 grams or ¾ oz of Whey Protein
5 grams or 0.18 oz of Walnuts

Protein 26g, Fat 8g, Carb 14g, Fibre 11g, 252 Kcals

Preparation

Place the nuts or seeds into the Tall Cup. Screw the Nutribullet Extractor Blade on to the top of the cup. Invert the cup, press it down into the Nutribullet Power Base and twist it into place. Blast them for 30 seconds. Put the rest of the solid ingredients into the cup and press them down below the Max Line. Add the fluid base to fill the cup up to the Max Line. Screw the Nutribullet Extractor Blade on to the top of the cup. Invert the cup, press it down into the Nutribullet Power Base and twist it into place. Blast the mixture until it is really smooth (20 or so seconds). *Enjoy!*

Lettuce and Guava Bonanza

Ingredients

1 Cup/Handful of Spinach (40 grams or 1½ oz)
1 Cup/Handful of Lettuce Leaves (40 grams or 1½ oz)
¾ Cup of Guava (90 grams or 3 oz)
¾ Cup of sliced Red Pepper (90 grams or 3 oz)
200 ml / 7 fl oz of Almond Milk (Unsweetened)
25 grams or ¾ oz of Whey Protein
4 grams or 0.14 oz of Pecans

Protein 25g, Fat 8g, Carb 15g, Fibre 12g, 253 Kcals

Preparation

Place the nuts or seeds into the Tall Cup. Screw the Nutribullet Extractor Blade on to the top of the cup. Invert the cup, press it down into the Nutribullet Power Base and twist it into place. Blast them for 30 seconds. Put the rest of the solid ingredients into the cup and press them down below the Max Line. Add the fluid base to fill the cup up to the Max Line. Screw the Nutribullet Extractor Blade on to the top of the cup. Invert the cup, press it down into the Nutribullet Power Base and twist it into place. Blast the mixture until it is really smooth (20 or so seconds). *Enjoy!*

Rocket hugs Nectarine

Ingredients

1 Cup/Handful of Broccoli Florets (40 grams or 1½ oz)
1 Cup/Handful of Rocket/Arugura Lettuce (40 grams or 1½ oz)
¾ Cup of Nectarine segments (90 grams or 3 oz)
¾ Cup of sliced Tomato (90 grams or 3 oz)
200 ml / 7 fl oz of Almond Milk (Unsweetened)
25 grams or ¾ oz of Rice Protein
11 grams or 0.39 oz of Flax Seeds

Protein 26g, Fat 8g, Carb 15g, Fibre 8g, 253 Kcals

Preparation

Place the nuts or seeds into the Tall Cup. Screw the Nutribullet Extractor Blade on to the top of the cup. Invert the cup, press it down into the Nutribullet Power Base and twist it into place. Blast them for 30 seconds. Put the rest of the solid ingredients into the cup and press them down below the Max Line. Add the fluid base to fill the cup up to the Max Line. Screw the Nutribullet Extractor Blade on to the top of the cup. Invert the cup, press it down into the Nutribullet Power Base and twist it into place. Blast the mixture until it is really smooth (20 or so seconds). *Enjoy!*

Raspberry joins Red Pepper

Ingredients

1 Cup/Handful of Rocket/Arugura Lettuce (40 grams or 1½ oz)
1 Cup/Handful of Broccoli Florets (40 grams or 1½ oz)
¾ Cup of Raspberries (90 grams or 3 oz)
¾ Cup of sliced Red Pepper (90 grams or 3 oz)
200 ml / 7 fl oz of Almond Milk (Unsweetened)
25 grams or ¾ oz of Whey Protein
8 grams or 0.28 oz of Chia Seeds

Protein 25g, Fat 7g, Carb 13g, Fibre 15g, 253 Kcals

Preparation

Place the nuts or seeds into the Tall Cup. Screw the Nutribullet Extractor Blade on to the top of the cup. Invert the cup, press it down into the Nutribullet Power Base and twist it into place. Blast them for 30 seconds. Put the rest of the solid ingredients into the cup and press them down below the Max Line. Add the fluid base to fill the cup up to the Max Line. Screw the Nutribullet Extractor Blade on to the top of the cup. Invert the cup, press it down into the Nutribullet Power Base and twist it into place. Blast the mixture until it is really smooth (20 or so seconds). *Enjoy!*

Blackberry Feast

Ingredients

1 Cup/Handful of Rocket/Arugura Lettuce (40 grams or 1½ oz)
1 Cup/Handful of Broccoli Florets (40 grams or 1½ oz)
¾ Cup of Blackberries (90 grams or 3 oz)
¾ Cup of sliced Tomato (90 grams or 3 oz)
200 ml / 7 fl oz of Almond Milk (Unsweetened)
25 grams or ¾ oz of Whey Protein
11 grams or 0.39 oz of Flax Seeds

Protein 26g, Fat 9g, Carb 11g, Fibre 13g, 253 Kcals

Preparation

Place the nuts or seeds into the Tall Cup. Screw the Nutribullet Extractor Blade on to the top of the cup. Invert the cup, press it down into the Nutribullet Power Base and twist it into place. Blast them for 30 seconds. Put the rest of the solid ingredients into the cup and press them down below the Max Line. Add the fluid base to fill the cup up to the Max Line. Screw the Nutribullet Extractor Blade on to the top of the cup. Invert the cup, press it down into the Nutribullet Power Base and twist it into place. Blast the mixture until it is really smooth (20 or so seconds). **Enjoy!**

Lettuce Elixir

Ingredients

1 Cup/Handful of Lettuce Leaves (40 grams or 1½ oz)
1 Cup/Handful of Rocket/Arugura Lettuce (40 grams or 1½ oz)
¾ Cup of Orange segments (90 grams or 3 oz)
¾ Cup of sliced Carrots (90 grams or 3 oz)
200 ml / 7 fl oz of Almond Milk (Unsweetened)
25 grams or ¾ oz of Pea Protein
7 grams or 0.25 oz of Chia Seeds

Protein 24g, Fat 6g, Carb 19g, Fibre 9g, 253 Kcals

Preparation

Place the nuts or seeds into the Tall Cup. Screw the Nutribullet Extractor Blade on to the top of the cup. Invert the cup, press it down into the Nutribullet Power Base and twist it into place. Blast them for 30 seconds. Put the rest of the solid ingredients into the cup and press them down below the Max Line. Add the fluid base to fill the cup up to the Max Line. Screw the Nutribullet Extractor Blade on to the top of the cup. Invert the cup, press it down into the Nutribullet Power Base and twist it into place. Blast the mixture until it is really smooth (20 or so seconds). **Enjoy!**

Lettuce and Nectarine Tonic

Ingredients

1 Cup/Handful of Spinach (40 grams or 1½ oz)
1 Cup/Handful of Lettuce Leaves (40 grams or 1½ oz)
¾ Cup of Nectarine segments (90 grams or 3 oz)
¾ Cup of sliced Red Pepper (90 grams or 3 oz)
200 ml / 7 fl oz of Almond Milk (Unsweetened)
25 grams or ¾ oz of Pea Protein
8 grams or 0.28 oz of Flax Seeds

Protein 25g, Fat 7g, Carb 16g, Fibre 8g, 253 Kcals

Preparation

Place the nuts or seeds into the Tall Cup. Screw the Nutribullet Extractor Blade on to the top of the cup. Invert the cup, press it down into the Nutribullet Power Base and twist it into place. Blast them for 30 seconds. Put the rest of the solid ingredients into the cup and press them down below the Max Line. Add the fluid base to fill the cup up to the Max Line. Screw the Nutribullet Extractor Blade on to the top of the cup. Invert the cup, press it down into the Nutribullet Power Base and twist it into place. Blast the mixture until it is really smooth (20 or so seconds). **Enjoy!**

Lettuce and Broccoli Machine

Ingredients

1 Cup/Handful of Lettuce Leaves (40 grams or 1½ oz)
1 Cup/Handful of Broccoli Florets (40 grams or 1½ oz)
¾ Cup of Blueberries (90 grams or 3 oz)
¾ Cup of sliced Tomato (90 grams or 3 oz)
200 ml / 7 fl oz of Almond Milk (Unsweetened)
22 grams or ¾ oz of Soy Protein
8 grams or 0.28 oz of Pecans

Protein 24g, Fat 9g, Carb 17g, Fibre 7g, 254 Kcals

Preparation

Place the nuts or seeds into the Tall Cup. Screw the Nutribullet Extractor Blade on to the top of the cup. Invert the cup, press it down into the Nutribullet Power Base and twist it into place. Blast them for 30 seconds. Put the rest of the solid ingredients into the cup and press them down below the Max Line. Add the fluid base to fill the cup up to the Max Line. Screw the Nutribullet Extractor Blade on to the top of the cup. Invert the cup, press it down into the Nutribullet Power Base and twist it into place. Blast the mixture until it is really smooth (20 or so seconds). **Enjoy!**

Nectarine Miracle

Ingredients

1 Cup/Handful of Spinach (40 grams or 1½ oz)
1 Cup/Handful of Broccoli Florets (40 grams or 1½ oz)
¾ Cup of Nectarine segments (90 grams or 3 oz)
¾ Cup of sliced Cauliflower florets (90 grams or 3 oz)
200 ml / 7 fl oz of Almond Milk (Unsweetened)
25 grams or ¾ oz of Pea Protein
7 grams or 0.25 oz of Sesame Seeds Hulled

Protein 27g, Fat 8g, Carb 16g, Fibre 7g, 254 Kcals

Preparation

Place the nuts or seeds into the Tall Cup. Screw the Nutribullet Extractor Blade on to the top of the cup. Invert the cup, press it down into the Nutribullet Power Base and twist it into place. Blast them for 30 seconds. Put the rest of the solid ingredients into the cup and press them down below the Max Line. Add the fluid base to fill the cup up to the Max Line. Screw the Nutribullet Extractor Blade on to the top of the cup. Invert the cup, press it down into the Nutribullet Power Base and twist it into place. Blast the mixture until it is really smooth (20 or so seconds). **Enjoy!**

Spinach and Blackberry Fix

Ingredients

1 Cup/Handful of Spinach (40 grams or 1½ oz)
1 Cup/Handful of Rocket/Arugura Lettuce (40 grams or 1½ oz)
¾ Cup of Blackberries (90 grams or 3 oz)
¾ Cup of sliced Red Pepper (90 grams or 3 oz)
200 ml / 7 fl oz of Almond Milk (Unsweetened)
25 grams or ¾ oz of Whey Protein
8 grams or 0.28 oz of Walnuts

Protein 25g, Fat 10g, Carb 11g, Fibre 11g, 254 Kcals

Preparation

Place the nuts or seeds into the Tall Cup. Screw the Nutribullet Extractor Blade on to the top of the cup. Invert the cup, press it down into the Nutribullet Power Base and twist it into place. Blast them for 30 seconds. Put the rest of the solid ingredients into the cup and press them down below the Max Line. Add the fluid base to fill the cup up to the Max Line. Screw the Nutribullet Extractor Blade on to the top of the cup. Invert the cup, press it down into the Nutribullet Power Base and twist it into place. Blast the mixture until it is really smooth (20 or so seconds). **Enjoy!**

Broccoli Orchard

Ingredients

1 Cup/Handful of Broccoli Florets (40 grams or 1½ oz)
1 Cup/Handful of Spinach (40 grams or 1½ oz)
¾ Cup of Blackberries (90 grams or 3 oz)
¾ Cup of sliced Carrots (90 grams or 3 oz)
200 ml / 7 fl oz of Almond Milk (Unsweetened)
25 grams or ¾ oz of Whey Protein
6 grams or 0.21 oz of Sesame Seeds Hulled

Protein 25g, Fat 8g, Carb 14g, Fibre 12g, 254 Kcals

Preparation

Place the nuts or seeds into the Tall Cup. Screw the Nutribullet Extractor Blade on to the top of the cup. Invert the cup, press it down into the Nutribullet Power Base and twist it into place. Blast them for 30 seconds. Put the rest of the solid ingredients into the cup and press them down below the Max Line. Add the fluid base to fill the cup up to the Max Line. Screw the Nutribullet Extractor Blade on to the top of the cup. Invert the cup, press it down into the Nutribullet Power Base and twist it into place. Blast the mixture until it is really smooth (20 or so seconds). **Enjoy!**

Lettuce and Orange Chorus

Ingredients

1 Cup/Handful of Lettuce Leaves (40 grams or 1½ oz)
1 Cup/Handful of Broccoli Florets (40 grams or 1½ oz)
¾ Cup of Orange segments (90 grams or 3 oz)
¾ Cup of sliced Carrots (90 grams or 3 oz)
200 ml / 7 fl oz of Almond Milk (Unsweetened)
25 grams or ¾ oz of Pea Protein
4 grams or 0.14 oz of Pecans

Protein 24g, Fat 6g, Carb 20g, Fibre 8g, 254 Kcals

Preparation

Place the nuts or seeds into the Tall Cup. Screw the Nutribullet Extractor Blade on to the top of the cup. Invert the cup, press it down into the Nutribullet Power Base and twist it into place. Blast them for 30 seconds. Put the rest of the solid ingredients into the cup and press them down below the Max Line. Add the fluid base to fill the cup up to the Max Line. Screw the Nutribullet Extractor Blade on to the top of the cup. Invert the cup, press it down into the Nutribullet Power Base and twist it into place. Blast the mixture until it is really smooth (20 or so seconds). **Enjoy!**

Blueberry and Tomato Concerto

Ingredients

2 Cups/Handfuls of Broccoli Florets (80 grams or 3 oz)
¾ Cup of Blueberries (90 grams or 3 oz)
¾ Cup of sliced Tomato (90 grams or 3 oz)
200 ml / 7 fl oz of Almond Milk (Unsweetened)
25 grams or ¾ oz of Pea Protein
5 grams or 0.18 oz of Walnuts

Protein 25g, Fat 7g, Carb 20g, Fibre 6g, 255 Kcals

Preparation

Place the nuts or seeds into the Tall Cup. Screw the Nutribullet Extractor Blade on to the top of the cup. Invert the cup, press it down into the Nutribullet Power Base and twist it into place. Blast them for 30 seconds. Put the rest of the solid ingredients into the cup and press them down below the Max Line. Add the fluid base to fill the cup up to the Max Line. Screw the Nutribullet Extractor Blade on to the top of the cup. Invert the cup, press it down into the Nutribullet Power Base and twist it into place. Blast the mixture until it is really smooth (20 or so seconds). ***Enjoy!***

Strawberry and Tomato Supermodel

Ingredients

1 Cup/Handful of Spinach (40 grams or 1½ oz)
1 Cup/Handful of Lettuce Leaves (40 grams or 1½ oz)
¾ Cup of Strawberries (90 grams or 3 oz)
¾ Cup of sliced Tomato (90 grams or 3 oz)
200 ml / 7 fl oz of Almond Milk (Unsweetened)
22 grams or ¾ oz of Soy Protein
14 grams or 0.49 oz of Sesame Seeds Hulled

Protein 26g, Fat 11g, Carb 10g, Fibre 7g, 255 Kcals

Preparation

Place the nuts or seeds into the Tall Cup. Screw the Nutribullet Extractor Blade on to the top of the cup. Invert the cup, press it down into the Nutribullet Power Base and twist it into place. Blast them for 30 seconds. Put the rest of the solid ingredients into the cup and press them down below the Max Line. Add the fluid base to fill the cup up to the Max Line. Screw the Nutribullet Extractor Blade on to the top of the cup. Invert the cup, press it down into the Nutribullet Power Base and twist it into place. Blast the mixture until it is really smooth (20 or so seconds). ***Enjoy!***

Carrot Medley

Ingredients

1 Cup/Handful of Lettuce Leaves (40 grams or 1½ oz)
1 Cup/Handful of Broccoli Florets (40 grams or 1½ oz)
¾ Cup of Raspberries (90 grams or 3 oz)
¾ Cup of sliced Carrots (90 grams or 3 oz)
200 ml / 7 fl oz of Almond Milk (Unsweetened)
25 grams or ¾ oz of Rice Protein
5 grams or 0.18 oz of Walnuts

Protein 25g, Fat 7g, Carb 16g, Fibre 11g, 256 Kcals

Preparation

Place the nuts or seeds into the Tall Cup. Screw the Nutribullet Extractor Blade on to the top of the cup. Invert the cup, press it down into the Nutribullet Power Base and twist it into place. Blast them for 30 seconds. Put the rest of the solid ingredients into the cup and press them down below the Max Line. Add the fluid base to fill the cup up to the Max Line. Screw the Nutribullet Extractor Blade on to the top of the cup. Invert the cup, press it down into the Nutribullet Power Base and twist it into place. Blast the mixture until it is really smooth (20 or so seconds). **Enjoy!**

Orange Dance

Ingredients

1 Cup/Handful of Rocket/Arugura Lettuce (40 grams or 1½ oz)
1 Cup/Handful of Spinach (40 grams or 1½ oz)
¾ Cup of Orange segments (90 grams or 3 oz)
¾ Cup of sliced Carrots (90 grams or 3 oz)
200 ml / 7 fl oz of Almond Milk (Unsweetened)
25 grams or ¾ oz of Pea Protein
5 grams or 0.18 oz of Pecans

Protein 24g, Fat 7g, Carb 19g, Fibre 7g, 256 Kcals

Preparation

Place the nuts or seeds into the Tall Cup. Screw the Nutribullet Extractor Blade on to the top of the cup. Invert the cup, press it down into the Nutribullet Power Base and twist it into place. Blast them for 30 seconds. Put the rest of the solid ingredients into the cup and press them down below the Max Line. Add the fluid base to fill the cup up to the Max Line. Screw the Nutribullet Extractor Blade on to the top of the cup. Invert the cup, press it down into the Nutribullet Power Base and twist it into place. Blast the mixture until it is really smooth (20 or so seconds). **Enjoy!**

Clear Thinking Brain Food
High in Omega3, Beta Carotene, Lycopene, Magnesium, Zinc, Vitamins B, C, E

Blackberry Fandango

Ingredients

1 Cup/Handful of Watercress (40 grams or 1½ oz)
1 Cup/Handful of Spinach (40 grams or 1½ oz)
¾ Cup of Blackberries (90 grams or 3 oz)
¾ Cup of Blueberries (90 grams or 3 oz)
200 ml / 7 fl oz of Coconut Milk
25 grams or ¾ oz of Rice Protein
2 grams or 0.07 oz of Pecans

Protein 24g, Fat 4g, Carb 24g, Fibre 8g, 250 Kcals

Preparation

Place the nuts or seeds into the Tall Cup. Screw the Nutribullet Extractor Blade on to the top of the cup. Invert the cup, press it down into the Nutribullet Power Base and twist it into place. Blast them for 30 seconds. Put the rest of the solid ingredients into the cup and press them down below the Max Line. Add the fluid base to fill the cup up to the Max Line. Screw the Nutribullet Extractor Blade on to the top of the cup. Invert the cup, press it down into the Nutribullet Power Base and twist it into place. Blast the mixture until it is really smooth (20 or so seconds). ***Enjoy!***

Mint embraces Blackberry

Ingredients

1 Cup/Handful of Spinach (40 grams or 1½ oz)
1 Cup/Handful of Mint (40 grams or 1½ oz)
¾ Cup of Strawberries (90 grams or 3 oz)
¾ Cup of Blackberries (90 grams or 3 oz)
200 ml / 7 fl oz of Water
25 grams or ¾ oz of Rice Protein
11 grams or 0.39 oz of Almonds

Protein 27g, Fat 7g, Carb 13g, Fibre 11g, 252 Kcals

Preparation

Place the nuts or seeds into the Tall Cup. Screw the Nutribullet Extractor Blade on to the top of the cup. Invert the cup, press it down into the Nutribullet Power Base and twist it into place. Blast them for 30 seconds. Put the rest of the solid ingredients into the cup and press them down below the Max Line. Add the fluid base to fill the cup up to the Max Line. Screw the Nutribullet Extractor Blade on to the top of the cup. Invert the cup, press it down into the Nutribullet Power Base and twist it into place. Blast the mixture until it is really smooth (20 or so seconds). ***Enjoy!***

Spinach hugs Strawberry

Ingredients

2 Cups/Handfuls of Spinach (80 grams or 3 oz)
¾ Cup of Blackberries (90 grams or 3 oz)
¾ Cup of Strawberries (90 grams or 3 oz)
200 ml / 7 fl oz of Water
22 grams or ¾ oz of Soy Protein
13 grams or 0.46 oz of Hazelnuts

Protein 26g, Fat 9g, Carb 12g, Fibre 10g, 252 Kcals

Preparation

Place the nuts or seeds into the Tall Cup. Screw the Nutribullet Extractor Blade on to the top of the cup. Invert the cup, press it down into the Nutribullet Power Base and twist it into place. Blast them for 30 seconds. Put the rest of the solid ingredients into the cup and press them down below the Max Line. Add the fluid base to fill the cup up to the Max Line. Screw the Nutribullet Extractor Blade on to the top of the cup. Invert the cup, press it down into the Nutribullet Power Base and twist it into place. Blast the mixture until it is really smooth (20 or so seconds). **Enjoy!**

Green Cabbage Surprise

Ingredients

1 Cup/Handful of Green Cabbage (40 grams or 1½ oz)
1 Cup/Handful of Mint (40 grams or 1½ oz)
1½ Cups of Blackberries (180 grams or 6 oz)
200 ml / 7 fl oz of Almond Milk (Unsweetened)
25 grams or ¾ oz of Whey Protein
5 grams or 0.18 oz of Cashews

Protein 25g, Fat 7g, Carb 13g, Fibre 16g, 253 Kcals

Preparation

Place the nuts or seeds into the Tall Cup. Screw the Nutribullet Extractor Blade on to the top of the cup. Invert the cup, press it down into the Nutribullet Power Base and twist it into place. Blast them for 30 seconds. Put the rest of the solid ingredients into the cup and press them down below the Max Line. Add the fluid base to fill the cup up to the Max Line. Screw the Nutribullet Extractor Blade on to the top of the cup. Invert the cup, press it down into the Nutribullet Power Base and twist it into place. Blast the mixture until it is really smooth (20 or so seconds). **Enjoy!**

Mint invites Blueberry

Ingredients

1 Cup/Handful of Bok Choy (40 grams or 1½ oz)
1 Cup/Handful of Mint (40 grams or 1½ oz)
1½ Cups of Blueberries (180 grams or 6 oz)
200 ml / 7 fl oz of Water
25 grams or ¾ oz of Rice Protein
6 grams or 0.21 oz of Sesame Seeds Hulled

Protein 24g, Fat 5g, Carb 25g, Fibre 8g, 254 Kcals

Preparation

Place the nuts or seeds into the Tall Cup. Screw the Nutribullet Extractor Blade on to the top of the cup. Invert the cup, press it down into the Nutribullet Power Base and twist it into place. Blast them for 30 seconds. Put the rest of the solid ingredients into the cup and press them down below the Max Line. Add the fluid base to fill the cup up to the Max Line. Screw the Nutribullet Extractor Blade on to the top of the cup. Invert the cup, press it down into the Nutribullet Power Base and twist it into place. Blast the mixture until it is really smooth (20 or so seconds). *Enjoy!*

Mint Sunrise

Ingredients

1 Cup/Handful of Mint (40 grams or 1½ oz)
1 Cup/Handful of Watercress (40 grams or 1½ oz)
¾ Cup of Blackberries (90 grams or 3 oz)
¾ Cup of sliced Carrots (90 grams or 3 oz)
200 ml / 7 fl oz of Coconut Milk
22 grams or ¾ oz of Soy Protein
5 grams or 0.18 oz of Almonds

Protein 25g, Fat 5g, Carb 18g, Fibre 11g, 252 Kcals

Preparation

Place the nuts or seeds into the Tall Cup. Screw the Nutribullet Extractor Blade on to the top of the cup. Invert the cup, press it down into the Nutribullet Power Base and twist it into place. Blast them for 30 seconds. Put the rest of the solid ingredients into the cup and press them down below the Max Line. Add the fluid base to fill the cup up to the Max Line. Screw the Nutribullet Extractor Blade on to the top of the cup. Invert the cup, press it down into the Nutribullet Power Base and twist it into place. Blast the mixture until it is really smooth (20 or so seconds). *Enjoy!*

Green Cabbage joins Blueberry

Ingredients

1 Cup/Handful of Green Cabbage (40 grams or 1½ oz)
1 Cup/Handful of Spinach (40 grams or 1½ oz)
¾ Cup of Blueberries (90 grams or 3 oz)
¾ Cup of sliced Tomato (90 grams or 3 oz)
200 ml / 7 fl oz of Hazelnut Milk
25 grams or ¾ oz of Pea Protein
1 gram or 0.04 oz of Walnuts

Protein 23g, Fat 5g, Carb 24g, Fibre 6g, 252 Kcals

Preparation

Place the nuts or seeds into the Tall Cup. Screw the Nutribullet Extractor Blade on to the top of the cup. Invert the cup, press it down into the Nutribullet Power Base and twist it into place. Blast them for 30 seconds. Put the rest of the solid ingredients into the cup and press them down below the Max Line. Add the fluid base to fill the cup up to the Max Line. Screw the Nutribullet Extractor Blade on to the top of the cup. Invert the cup, press it down into the Nutribullet Power Base and twist it into place. Blast the mixture until it is really smooth (20 or so seconds). *Enjoy!*

Rocket and Green Cabbage Waterfall

Ingredients

1 Cup/Handful of Rocket/Arugura Lettuce (40 grams or 1½ oz)
1 Cup/Handful of Green Cabbage (40 grams or 1½ oz)
¾ Cup of Blueberries (90 grams or 3 oz)
¾ Cup of sliced Tomato (90 grams or 3 oz)
200 ml / 7 fl oz of Water
25 grams or ¾ oz of Pea Protein
10 grams or 0.35 oz of Pecans

Protein 23g, Fat 9g, Carb 18g, Fibre 6g, 254 Kcals

Preparation

Place the nuts or seeds into the Tall Cup. Screw the Nutribullet Extractor Blade on to the top of the cup. Invert the cup, press it down into the Nutribullet Power Base and twist it into place. Blast them for 30 seconds. Put the rest of the solid ingredients into the cup and press them down below the Max Line. Add the fluid base to fill the cup up to the Max Line. Screw the Nutribullet Extractor Blade on to the top of the cup. Invert the cup, press it down into the Nutribullet Power Base and twist it into place. Blast the mixture until it is really smooth (20 or so seconds). *Enjoy!*

Watercress meets Strawberry

Ingredients

2 Cups/Handfuls of Watercress (80 grams or 3 oz)
¾ Cup of Strawberries (90 grams or 3 oz)
¾ Cup of sliced Tomato (90 grams or 3 oz)
200 ml / 7 fl oz of Coconut Milk
25 grams or ¾ oz of Rice Protein
12 grams or 0.42 oz of Pumpkin Seeds

Protein 26g, Fat 8g, Carb 17g, Fibre 4g, 254 Kcals

Preparation

Place the nuts or seeds into the Tall Cup. Screw the Nutribullet Extractor Blade on to the top of the cup. Invert the cup, press it down into the Nutribullet Power Base and twist it into place. Blast them for 30 seconds. Put the rest of the solid ingredients into the cup and press them down below the Max Line. Add the fluid base to fill the cup up to the Max Line. Screw the Nutribullet Extractor Blade on to the top of the cup. Invert the cup, press it down into the Nutribullet Power Base and twist it into place. Blast the mixture until it is really smooth (20 or so seconds). **Enjoy!**

Spinach and Strawberry Blossom

Ingredients

1 Cup/Handful of Bok Choy (40 grams or 1½ oz)
1 Cup/Handful of Spinach (40 grams or 1½ oz)
¾ Cup of Strawberries (90 grams or 3 oz)
¾ Cup of sliced Tomato (90 grams or 3 oz)
200 ml / 7 fl oz of Almond Milk (Unsweetened)
25 grams or ¾ oz of Whey Protein
12 grams or 0.42 oz of Hazelnuts

Protein 25g, Fat 11g, Carb 12g, Fibre 8g, 255 Kcals

Preparation

Place the nuts or seeds into the Tall Cup. Screw the Nutribullet Extractor Blade on to the top of the cup. Invert the cup, press it down into the Nutribullet Power Base and twist it into place. Blast them for 30 seconds. Put the rest of the solid ingredients into the cup and press them down below the Max Line. Add the fluid base to fill the cup up to the Max Line. Screw the Nutribullet Extractor Blade on to the top of the cup. Invert the cup, press it down into the Nutribullet Power Base and twist it into place. Blast the mixture until it is really smooth (20 or so seconds). **Enjoy!**

Happiness, Deep Sleep and Stress Busters
High in Tryptophan, Magnesium, Vit B3, B6, B9

Carrot Extracted

Ingredients

1 Cup/Handful of Spinach (40 grams or 1½ oz)
1 Cup/Handful of Broccoli Florets (40 grams or 1½ oz)
¾ Cup of Apricot halves (90 grams or 3 oz)
¾ Cup of sliced Carrots (90 grams or 3 oz)
200 ml / 7 fl oz of Almond Milk (Unsweetened)
25 grams or ¾ oz of Pea Protein
4 grams or 0.14 oz of Chia Seeds

Protein 25g, Fat 5g, Carb 20g, Fibre 8g, 250 Kcals

Preparation

Place the nuts or seeds into the Tall Cup. Screw the Nutribullet Extractor Blade on to the top of the cup. Invert the cup, press it down into the Nutribullet Power Base and twist it into place. Blast them for 30 seconds. Put the rest of the solid ingredients into the cup and press them down below the Max Line. Add the fluid base to fill the cup up to the Max Line. Screw the Nutribullet Extractor Blade on to the top of the cup. Invert the cup, press it down into the Nutribullet Power Base and twist it into place. Blast the mixture until it is really smooth (20 or so seconds). ***Enjoy!***

Cauliflower Dance

Ingredients

1 Cup/Handful of Broccoli Florets (40 grams or 1½ oz)
1 Cup/Handful of Watercress (40 grams or 1½ oz)
¾ Cup of Apricot halves (90 grams or 3 oz)
¾ Cup of sliced Cauliflower florets (90 grams or 3 oz)
200 ml / 7 fl oz of Almond Milk (Unsweetened)
22 grams or ¾ oz of Soy Protein
10 grams or 0.35 oz of Cashews

Protein 27g, Fat 7g, Carb 17g, Fibre 6g, 250 Kcals

Preparation

Place the nuts or seeds into the Tall Cup. Screw the Nutribullet Extractor Blade on to the top of the cup. Invert the cup, press it down into the Nutribullet Power Base and twist it into place. Blast them for 30 seconds. Put the rest of the solid ingredients into the cup and press them down below the Max Line. Add the fluid base to fill the cup up to the Max Line. Screw the Nutribullet Extractor Blade on to the top of the cup. Invert the cup, press it down into the Nutribullet Power Base and twist it into place. Blast the mixture until it is really smooth (20 or so seconds). ***Enjoy!***

Apricot Royale

Ingredients

1 Cup/Handful of Watercress (40 grams or 1½ oz)
1 Cup/Handful of Spinach (40 grams or 1½ oz)
¾ Cup of Apricot halves (90 grams or 3 oz)
¾ Cup of sliced Cauliflower florets (90 grams or 3 oz)
200 ml / 7 fl oz of Almond Milk (Unsweetened)
25 grams or ¾ oz of Whey Protein
10 grams or 0.35 oz of Sunflower Seeds Hulled

Protein 27g, Fat 9g, Carb 15g, Fibre 8g, 251 Kcals

Preparation

Place the nuts or seeds into the Tall Cup. Screw the Nutribullet Extractor Blade on to the top of the cup. Invert the cup, press it down into the Nutribullet Power Base and twist it into place. Blast them for 30 seconds. Put the rest of the solid ingredients into the cup and press them down below the Max Line. Add the fluid base to fill the cup up to the Max Line. Screw the Nutribullet Extractor Blade on to the top of the cup. Invert the cup, press it down into the Nutribullet Power Base and twist it into place. Blast the mixture until it is really smooth (20 or so seconds). **Enjoy!**

Spinach and Apricot Cornucopia

Ingredients

2 Cups/Handfuls of Spinach (80 grams or 3 oz)
¾ Cup of Apricot halves (90 grams or 3 oz)
¾ Cup of sliced Fine Beans (90 grams or 3 oz)
200 ml / 7 fl oz of Almond Milk (Unsweetened)
22 grams or ¾ oz of Soy Protein
10 grams or 0.35 oz of Pumpkin Seeds

Protein 28g, Fat 8g, Carb 15g, Fibre 7g, 251 Kcals

Preparation

Place the nuts or seeds into the Tall Cup. Screw the Nutribullet Extractor Blade on to the top of the cup. Invert the cup, press it down into the Nutribullet Power Base and twist it into place. Blast them for 30 seconds. Put the rest of the solid ingredients into the cup and press them down below the Max Line. Add the fluid base to fill the cup up to the Max Line. Screw the Nutribullet Extractor Blade on to the top of the cup. Invert the cup, press it down into the Nutribullet Power Base and twist it into place. Blast the mixture until it is really smooth (20 or so seconds). **Enjoy!**

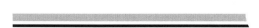

Spinach kisses Apricot

Ingredients

1 Cup/Handful of Spinach (40 grams or 1½ oz)
1 Cup/Handful of Watercress (40 grams or 1½ oz)
¾ Cup of Apricot halves (90 grams or 3 oz)
¾ Cup of sliced Carrots (90 grams or 3 oz)
200 ml / 7 fl oz of Almond Milk (Unsweetened)
25 grams or ¾ oz of Pea Protein
6 grams or 0.21 oz of Sunflower Seeds Hulled

Protein 26g, Fat 7g, Carb 19g, Fibre 7g, 252 Kcals

Preparation

Place the nuts or seeds into the Tall Cup. Screw the Nutribullet Extractor Blade on to the top of the cup. Invert the cup, press it down into the Nutribullet Power Base and twist it into place. Blast them for 30 seconds. Put the rest of the solid ingredients into the cup and press them down below the Max Line. Add the fluid base to fill the cup up to the Max Line. Screw the Nutribullet Extractor Blade on to the top of the cup. Invert the cup, press it down into the Nutribullet Power Base and twist it into place. Blast the mixture until it is really smooth (20 or so seconds). *Enjoy!*

Fine Bean Sensation

Ingredients

1 Cup/Handful of Spinach (40 grams or 1½ oz)
1 Cup/Handful of Watercress (40 grams or 1½ oz)
¾ Cup of Apricot halves (90 grams or 3 oz)
¾ Cup of sliced Fine Beans (90 grams or 3 oz)
200 ml / 7 fl oz of Almond Milk (Unsweetened)
22 grams or ¾ oz of Soy Protein
13 grams or 0.46 oz of Chia Seeds

Protein 28g, Fat 7g, Carb 14g, Fibre 10g, 253 Kcals

Preparation

Place the nuts or seeds into the Tall Cup. Screw the Nutribullet Extractor Blade on to the top of the cup. Invert the cup, press it down into the Nutribullet Power Base and twist it into place. Blast them for 30 seconds. Put the rest of the solid ingredients into the cup and press them down below the Max Line. Add the fluid base to fill the cup up to the Max Line. Screw the Nutribullet Extractor Blade on to the top of the cup. Invert the cup, press it down into the Nutribullet Power Base and twist it into place. Blast the mixture until it is really smooth (20 or so seconds). *Enjoy!*

Broccoli meets Apricot

Ingredients

2 Cups/Handfuls of Broccoli Florets (80 grams or 3 oz)
¾ Cup of Apricot halves (90 grams or 3 oz)
¾ Cup of sliced Fine Beans (90 grams or 3 oz)
200 ml / 7 fl oz of Almond Milk (Unsweetened)
25 grams or ¾ oz of Pea Protein
6 grams or 0.21 oz of Peanuts

Protein 27g, Fat 7g, Carb 18g, Fibre 7g, 254 Kcals

Preparation

Place the nuts or seeds into the Tall Cup. Screw the Nutribullet Extractor Blade on to the top of the cup. Invert the cup, press it down into the Nutribullet Power Base and twist it into place. Blast them for 30 seconds. Put the rest of the solid ingredients into the cup and press them down below the Max Line. Add the fluid base to fill the cup up to the Max Line. Screw the Nutribullet Extractor Blade on to the top of the cup. Invert the cup, press it down into the Nutribullet Power Base and twist it into place. Blast the mixture until it is really smooth (20 or so seconds). **Enjoy!**

Spinach Blend

Ingredients

2 Cups/Handfuls of Spinach (80 grams or 3 oz)
¾ Cup of Apricot halves (90 grams or 3 oz)
¾ Cup of sliced Carrots (90 grams or 3 oz)
200 ml / 7 fl oz of Almond Milk (Unsweetened)
25 grams or ¾ oz of Whey Protein
6 grams or 0.21 oz of Sesame Seeds Hulled

Protein 25g, Fat 8g, Carb 18g, Fibre 9g, 254 Kcals

Preparation

Place the nuts or seeds into the Tall Cup. Screw the Nutribullet Extractor Blade on to the top of the cup. Invert the cup, press it down into the Nutribullet Power Base and twist it into place. Blast them for 30 seconds. Put the rest of the solid ingredients into the cup and press them down below the Max Line. Add the fluid base to fill the cup up to the Max Line. Screw the Nutribullet Extractor Blade on to the top of the cup. Invert the cup, press it down into the Nutribullet Power Base and twist it into place. Blast the mixture until it is really smooth (20 or so seconds). **Enjoy!**

Beetroot Dictator

Ingredients

1 Cup/Handful of Broccoli Florets (40 grams or 1½ oz)
1 Cup/Handful of Watercress (40 grams or 1½ oz)
¾ Cup of Apricot halves (90 grams or 3 oz)
¾ Cup of diced Beetroot (90 grams or 3 oz)
200 ml / 7 fl oz of Almond Milk (Unsweetened)
25 grams or ¾ oz of Pea Protein
5 grams or 0.18 oz of Cashews

Protein 26g, Fat 6g, Carb 21g, Fibre 7g, 255 Kcals

Preparation

Place the nuts or seeds into the Tall Cup. Screw the Nutribullet Extractor Blade on to the top of the cup. Invert the cup, press it down into the Nutribullet Power Base and twist it into place. Blast them for 30 seconds. Put the rest of the solid ingredients into the cup and press them down below the Max Line. Add the fluid base to fill the cup up to the Max Line. Screw the Nutribullet Extractor Blade on to the top of the cup. Invert the cup, press it down into the Nutribullet Power Base and twist it into place. Blast the mixture until it is really smooth (20 or so seconds). **Enjoy!**

Watercress Concerto

Ingredients

2 Cups/Handfuls of Watercress (80 grams or 3 oz)
¾ Cup of Apricot halves (90 grams or 3 oz)
¾ Cup of sliced Carrots (90 grams or 3 oz)
200 ml / 7 fl oz of Almond Milk (Unsweetened)
25 grams or ¾ oz of Pea Protein
6 grams or 0.21 oz of Walnuts

Protein 25g, Fat 8g, Carb 18g, Fibre 6g, 255 Kcals

Preparation

Place the nuts or seeds into the Tall Cup. Screw the Nutribullet Extractor Blade on to the top of the cup. Invert the cup, press it down into the Nutribullet Power Base and twist it into place. Blast them for 30 seconds. Put the rest of the solid ingredients into the cup and press them down below the Max Line. Add the fluid base to fill the cup up to the Max Line. Screw the Nutribullet Extractor Blade on to the top of the cup. Invert the cup, press it down into the Nutribullet Power Base and twist it into place. Blast the mixture until it is really smooth (20 or so seconds). **Enjoy!**

5:2 Diet High Protein Specials

Pineapple and Tomato Cocktail

Ingredients

1 Cup/Handful of Bok Choy (40 grams or 1½ oz)
1 Cup/Handful of Green Cabbage (40 grams or 1½ oz)
¾ Cup of Pineapple chunks (90 grams or 3 oz)
¾ Cup of sliced Tomato (90 grams or 3 oz)
200 ml / 7 fl oz of Water
22 grams or ¾ oz of Soy Protein
15 grams or 0.53 oz of Almonds

Protein 25g, Fat 8g, Carb 17g, Fibre 5g, 250 Kcals

Preparation

Place the nuts or seeds into the Tall Cup. Screw the Nutribullet Extractor Blade on to the top of the cup. Invert the cup, press it down into the Nutribullet Power Base and twist it into place. Blast them for 30 seconds. Put the rest of the solid ingredients into the cup and press them down below the Max Line. Add the fluid base to fill the cup up to the Max Line. Screw the Nutribullet Extractor Blade on to the top of the cup. Invert the cup, press it down into the Nutribullet Power Base and twist it into place. Blast the mixture until it is really smooth (20 or so seconds). **Enjoy!**

Bok Choy and Apple Energizer

Ingredients

1 Cup/Handful of Bok Choy (40 grams or 1½ oz)
1 Cup/Handful of Fennel (40 grams or 1½ oz)
¾ Cup of Apple slices (90 grams or 3 oz)
¾ Cup of sliced Carrots (90 grams or 3 oz)
200 ml / 7 fl oz of Almond Milk (Unsweetened)
25 grams or ¾ oz of Whey Protein
5 grams or 0.18 oz of Pumpkin Seeds

Protein 23g, Fat 6g, Carb 21g, Fibre 9g, 250 Kcals

Preparation

Place the nuts or seeds into the Tall Cup. Screw the Nutribullet Extractor Blade on to the top of the cup. Invert the cup, press it down into the Nutribullet Power Base and twist it into place. Blast them for 30 seconds. Put the rest of the solid ingredients into the cup and press them down below the Max Line. Add the fluid base to fill the cup up to the Max Line. Screw the Nutribullet Extractor Blade on to the top of the cup. Invert the cup, press it down into the Nutribullet Power Base and twist it into place. Blast the mixture until it is really smooth (20 or so seconds). **Enjoy!**

Apple and Red Pepper Miracle

Ingredients

1 Cup/Handful of Bok Choy (40 grams or 1½ oz)
1 Cup/Handful of Red or White Cabbage (40 grams or 1½ oz)
¾ Cup of Apple slices (90 grams or 3 oz)
¾ Cup of sliced Red Pepper (90 grams or 3 oz)
200 ml / 7 fl oz of Hazelnut Milk
25 grams or ¾ oz of Rice Protein
1 gram or 0.04 oz of Brazil nuts

Protein 23g, Fat 5g, Carb 25g, Fibre 6g, 250 Kcals

Preparation

Place the nuts or seeds into the Tall Cup. Screw the Nutribullet Extractor Blade on to the top of the cup. Invert the cup, press it down into the Nutribullet Power Base and twist it into place. Blast them for 30 seconds. Put the rest of the solid ingredients into the cup and press them down below the Max Line. Add the fluid base to fill the cup up to the Max Line. Screw the Nutribullet Extractor Blade on to the top of the cup. Invert the cup, press it down into the Nutribullet Power Base and twist it into place. Blast the mixture until it is really smooth (20 or so seconds). *Enjoy!*

Celeriac Fandango

Ingredients

1 Cup/Handful of Fennel (40 grams or 1½ oz)
1 Cup/Handful of Watercress (40 grams or 1½ oz)
¾ Cup of Raspberries (90 grams or 3 oz)
¾ Cup of diced Celeriac (90 grams or 3 oz)
200 ml / 7 fl oz of Almond Milk (Unsweetened)
25 grams or ¾ oz of Rice Protein
5 grams or 0.18 oz of Almonds

Protein 26g, Fat 6g, Carb 17g, Fibre 10g, 250 Kcals

Preparation

Place the nuts or seeds into the Tall Cup. Screw the Nutribullet Extractor Blade on to the top of the cup. Invert the cup, press it down into the Nutribullet Power Base and twist it into place. Blast them for 30 seconds. Put the rest of the solid ingredients into the cup and press them down below the Max Line. Add the fluid base to fill the cup up to the Max Line. Screw the Nutribullet Extractor Blade on to the top of the cup. Invert the cup, press it down into the Nutribullet Power Base and twist it into place. Blast the mixture until it is really smooth (20 or so seconds). *Enjoy!*

Lettuce meets Apricot

Ingredients

2 Cups/Handfuls of Lettuce Leaves (80 grams or 3 oz)
¾ Cup of Apricot halves (90 grams or 3 oz)
¾ Cup of sliced Yellow Pepper (90 grams or 3 oz)
200 ml / 7 fl oz of Coconut Milk
22 grams or ¾ oz of Soy Protein
7 grams or 0.25 oz of Hazelnuts

Protein 24g, Fat 7g, Carb 20g, Fibre 5g, 250 Kcals

Preparation

Place the nuts or seeds into the Tall Cup. Screw the Nutribullet Extractor Blade on to the top of the cup. Invert the cup, press it down into the Nutribullet Power Base and twist it into place. Blast them for 30 seconds. Put the rest of the solid ingredients into the cup and press them down below the Max Line. Add the fluid base to fill the cup up to the Max Line. Screw the Nutribullet Extractor Blade on to the top of the cup. Invert the cup, press it down into the Nutribullet Power Base and twist it into place. Blast the mixture until it is really smooth (20 or so seconds). **Enjoy!**

Apple Dictator

Ingredients

1 Cup/Handful of Bok Choy (40 grams or 1½ oz)
1 Cup/Handful of Spinach (40 grams or 1½ oz)
¾ Cup of Apple slices (90 grams or 3 oz)
¾ Cup of sliced Carrots (90 grams or 3 oz)
200 ml / 7 fl oz of Coconut Milk
25 grams or ¾ oz of Pea Protein
2 grams or 0.07 oz of Sunflower Seeds Hulled

Protein 23g, Fat 4g, Carb 26g, Fibre 6g, 250 Kcals

Preparation

Place the nuts or seeds into the Tall Cup. Screw the Nutribullet Extractor Blade on to the top of the cup. Invert the cup, press it down into the Nutribullet Power Base and twist it into place. Blast them for 30 seconds. Put the rest of the solid ingredients into the cup and press them down below the Max Line. Add the fluid base to fill the cup up to the Max Line. Screw the Nutribullet Extractor Blade on to the top of the cup. Invert the cup, press it down into the Nutribullet Power Base and twist it into place. Blast the mixture until it is really smooth (20 or so seconds). **Enjoy!**

Broccoli embraces Green Cabbage

Ingredients

1 Cup/Handful of Broccoli Florets (40 grams or 1½ oz)
1 Cup/Handful of Green Cabbage (40 grams or 1½ oz)
¾ Cup of Papaya (90 grams or 3 oz)
¾ Cup of sliced Tomato (90 grams or 3 oz)
200 ml / 7 fl oz of Water
25 grams or ¾ oz of Rice Protein
12 grams or 0.42 oz of Walnuts

Protein 25g, Fat 9g, Carb 17g, Fibre 5g, 250 Kcals

Preparation

Place the nuts or seeds into the Tall Cup. Screw the Nutribullet Extractor Blade on to the top of the cup. Invert the cup, press it down into the Nutribullet Power Base and twist it into place. Blast them for 30 seconds. Put the rest of the solid ingredients into the cup and press them down below the Max Line. Add the fluid base to fill the cup up to the Max Line. Screw the Nutribullet Extractor Blade on to the top of the cup. Invert the cup, press it down into the Nutribullet Power Base and twist it into place. Blast the mixture until it is really smooth (20 or so seconds). **Enjoy!**

Grapefruit Delusion

Ingredients

2 Cups/Handfuls of Mint (80 grams or 3 oz)
¾ Cup of Grapefruit segments (90 grams or 3 oz)
¾ Cup of diced Celeriac (90 grams or 3 oz)
200 ml / 7 fl oz of Hazelnut Milk
22 grams or ¾ oz of Soy Protein
1 gram or 0.04 oz of Flax Seeds

Protein 25g, Fat 5g, Carb 21g, Fibre 9g, 250 Kcals

Preparation

Place the nuts or seeds into the Tall Cup. Screw the Nutribullet Extractor Blade on to the top of the cup. Invert the cup, press it down into the Nutribullet Power Base and twist it into place. Blast them for 30 seconds. Put the rest of the solid ingredients into the cup and press them down below the Max Line. Add the fluid base to fill the cup up to the Max Line. Screw the Nutribullet Extractor Blade on to the top of the cup. Invert the cup, press it down into the Nutribullet Power Base and twist it into place. Blast the mixture until it is really smooth (20 or so seconds). **Enjoy!**

Guava Fantasy

Ingredients

1 Cup/Handful of Rocket/Arugura Lettuce (40 grams or 1½ oz)
1 Cup/Handful of Green Cabbage (40 grams or 1½ oz)
¾ Cup of Guava (90 grams or 3 oz)
¾ Cup of sliced Cauliflower florets (90 grams or 3 oz)
200 ml / 7 fl oz of Almond Milk (Unsweetened)
25 grams or ¾ oz of Rice Protein
5 grams or 0.18 oz of Hazelnuts

Protein 27g, Fat 7g, Carb 16g, Fibre 9g, 250 Kcals

Preparation

Place the nuts or seeds into the Tall Cup. Screw the Nutribullet Extractor Blade on to the top of the cup. Invert the cup, press it down into the Nutribullet Power Base and twist it into place. Blast them for 30 seconds. Put the rest of the solid ingredients into the cup and press them down below the Max Line. Add the fluid base to fill the cup up to the Max Line. Screw the Nutribullet Extractor Blade on to the top of the cup. Invert the cup, press it down into the Nutribullet Power Base and twist it into place. Blast the mixture until it is really smooth (20 or so seconds). **Enjoy!**

Pear and Yellow Pepper Blockbuster

Ingredients

2 Cups/Handfuls of Spinach (80 grams or 3 oz)
¾ Cup of Pear slices (90 grams or 3 oz)
¾ Cup of sliced Yellow Pepper (90 grams or 3 oz)
200 ml / 7 fl oz of Hazelnut Milk
25 grams or ¾ oz of Rice Protein
1 gram or 0.04 oz of Sunflower Seeds Hulled

Protein 24g, Fat 5g, Carb 26g, Fibre 6g, 250 Kcals

Preparation

Place the nuts or seeds into the Tall Cup. Screw the Nutribullet Extractor Blade on to the top of the cup. Invert the cup, press it down into the Nutribullet Power Base and twist it into place. Blast them for 30 seconds. Put the rest of the solid ingredients into the cup and press them down below the Max Line. Add the fluid base to fill the cup up to the Max Line. Screw the Nutribullet Extractor Blade on to the top of the cup. Invert the cup, press it down into the Nutribullet Power Base and twist it into place. Blast the mixture until it is really smooth (20 or so seconds). **Enjoy!**

Green Cabbage and Bok Choy Paradox

Ingredients

1 Cup/Handful of Green Cabbage (40 grams or 1½ oz)
1 Cup/Handful of Bok Choy (40 grams or 1½ oz)
¾ Cup of Plum halves (90 grams or 3 oz)
¾ Cup of sliced Celery (90 grams or 3 oz)
200 ml / 7 fl oz of Coconut Milk
25 grams or ¾ oz of Pea Protein
6 grams or 0.21 oz of Hazelnuts

Protein 23g, Fat 7g, Carb 21g, Fibre 5g, 250 Kcals

Preparation

Place the nuts or seeds into the Tall Cup. Screw the Nutribullet Extractor Blade on to the top of the cup. Invert the cup, press it down into the Nutribullet Power Base and twist it into place. Blast them for 30 seconds. Put the rest of the solid ingredients into the cup and press them down below the Max Line. Add the fluid base to fill the cup up to the Max Line. Screw the Nutribullet Extractor Blade on to the top of the cup. Invert the cup, press it down into the Nutribullet Power Base and twist it into place. Blast the mixture until it is really smooth (20 or so seconds). *Enjoy!*

Raspberry and Celery Paradise

Ingredients

2 Cups/Handfuls of Watercress (80 grams or 3 oz)
¾ Cup of Raspberries (90 grams or 3 oz)
¾ Cup of sliced Celery (90 grams or 3 oz)
200 ml / 7 fl oz of Coconut Milk
25 grams or ¾ oz of Rice Protein
8 grams or 0.28 oz of Almonds

Protein 25g, Fat 7g, Carb 15g, Fibre 9g, 250 Kcals

Preparation

Place the nuts or seeds into the Tall Cup. Screw the Nutribullet Extractor Blade on to the top of the cup. Invert the cup, press it down into the Nutribullet Power Base and twist it into place. Blast them for 30 seconds. Put the rest of the solid ingredients into the cup and press them down below the Max Line. Add the fluid base to fill the cup up to the Max Line. Screw the Nutribullet Extractor Blade on to the top of the cup. Invert the cup, press it down into the Nutribullet Power Base and twist it into place. Blast the mixture until it is really smooth (20 or so seconds). *Enjoy!*

Apricot and Carrot Sunshine

Ingredients

2 Cups/Handfuls of Spinach (80 grams or 3 oz)
¾ Cup of Apricot halves (90 grams or 3 oz)
¾ Cup of sliced Carrots (90 grams or 3 oz)
200 ml / 7 fl oz of Almond Milk (Unsweetened)
25 grams or ¾ oz of Rice Protein
5 grams or 0.18 oz of Walnuts

Protein 26g, Fat 7g, Carb 19g, Fibre 7g, 250 Kcals

Preparation

Place the nuts or seeds into the Tall Cup. Screw the Nutribullet Extractor Blade on to the top of the cup. Invert the cup, press it down into the Nutribullet Power Base and twist it into place. Blast them for 30 seconds. Put the rest of the solid ingredients into the cup and press them down below the Max Line. Add the fluid base to fill the cup up to the Max Line. Screw the Nutribullet Extractor Blade on to the top of the cup. Invert the cup, press it down into the Nutribullet Power Base and twist it into place. Blast the mixture until it is really smooth (20 or so seconds). **Enjoy!**

Turnip Sunrise

Ingredients

2 Cups/Handfuls of Green Cabbage (80 grams or 3 oz)
¾ Cup of Clementine slices (90 grams or 3 oz)
¾ Cup of diced Turnip (90 grams or 3 oz)
200 ml / 7 fl oz of Almond Milk (Unsweetened)
25 grams or ¾ oz of Rice Protein
9 grams or 0.32 oz of Chia Seeds

Protein 25g, Fat 6g, Carb 19g, Fibre 9g, 250 Kcals

Preparation

Place the nuts or seeds into the Tall Cup. Screw the Nutribullet Extractor Blade on to the top of the cup. Invert the cup, press it down into the Nutribullet Power Base and twist it into place. Blast them for 30 seconds. Put the rest of the solid ingredients into the cup and press them down below the Max Line. Add the fluid base to fill the cup up to the Max Line. Screw the Nutribullet Extractor Blade on to the top of the cup. Invert the cup, press it down into the Nutribullet Power Base and twist it into place. Blast the mixture until it is really smooth (20 or so seconds). **Enjoy!**

Mint and Mango Vortex

Ingredients

1 Cup/Handful of Fennel (40 grams or 1½ oz)
1 Cup/Handful of Mint (40 grams or 1½ oz)
¾ Cup of Mango slices (90 grams or 3 oz)
¾ Cup of diced Turnip (90 grams or 3 oz)
200 ml / 7 fl oz of Water
25 grams or ¾ oz of Pea Protein
7 grams or 0.25 oz of Pumpkin Seeds

Protein 25g, Fat 5g, Carb 22g, Fibre 7g, 250 Kcals

Preparation

Place the nuts or seeds into the Tall Cup. Screw the Nutribullet Extractor Blade on to the top of the cup. Invert the cup, press it down into the Nutribullet Power Base and twist it into place. Blast them for 30 seconds. Put the rest of the solid ingredients into the cup and press them down below the Max Line. Add the fluid base to fill the cup up to the Max Line. Screw the Nutribullet Extractor Blade on to the top of the cup. Invert the cup, press it down into the Nutribullet Power Base and twist it into place. Blast the mixture until it is really smooth (20 or so seconds). **Enjoy!**

Spinach befriends Raspberry

Ingredients

1 Cup/Handful of Rocket/Arugura Lettuce (40 grams or 1½ oz)
1 Cup/Handful of Spinach (40 grams or 1½ oz)
¾ Cup of Raspberries (90 grams or 3 oz)
¾ Cup of Radishes (90 grams or 3 oz)
200 ml / 7 fl oz of Coconut Milk
25 grams or ¾ oz of Whey Protein
7 grams or 0.25 oz of Peanuts

Protein 24g, Fat 7g, Carb 16g, Fibre 11g, 250 Kcals

Preparation

Place the nuts or seeds into the Tall Cup. Screw the Nutribullet Extractor Blade on to the top of the cup. Invert the cup, press it down into the Nutribullet Power Base and twist it into place. Blast them for 30 seconds. Put the rest of the solid ingredients into the cup and press them down below the Max Line. Add the fluid base to fill the cup up to the Max Line. Screw the Nutribullet Extractor Blade on to the top of the cup. Invert the cup, press it down into the Nutribullet Power Base and twist it into place. Blast the mixture until it is really smooth (20 or so seconds). **Enjoy!**

Broccoli hugs Blackberry

Ingredients

1 Cup/Handful of Rocket/Arugura Lettuce (40 grams or 1½ oz)
1 Cup/Handful of Broccoli Florets (40 grams or 1½ oz)
¾ Cup of Blackberries (90 grams or 3 oz)
¾ Cup of sliced Tomato (90 grams or 3 oz)
200 ml / 7 fl oz of Hazelnut Milk
25 grams or ¾ oz of Whey Protein
4 grams or 0.14 oz of Almonds

Protein 24g, Fat 7g, Carb 17g, Fibre 10g, 250 Kcals

Preparation

Place the nuts or seeds into the Tall Cup. Screw the Nutribullet Extractor Blade on to the top of the cup. Invert the cup, press it down into the Nutribullet Power Base and twist it into place. Blast them for 30 seconds. Put the rest of the solid ingredients into the cup and press them down below the Max Line. Add the fluid base to fill the cup up to the Max Line. Screw the Nutribullet Extractor Blade on to the top of the cup. Invert the cup, press it down into the Nutribullet Power Base and twist it into place. Blast the mixture until it is really smooth (20 or so seconds). **Enjoy!**

Fennel partners Broccoli

Ingredients

1 Cup/Handful of Fennel (40 grams or 1½ oz)
1 Cup/Handful of Broccoli Florets (40 grams or 1½ oz)
¾ Cup of Melon chunks (90 grams or 3 oz)
¾ Cup of diced Turnip (90 grams or 3 oz)
200 ml / 7 fl oz of Almond Milk (Unsweetened)
25 grams or ¾ oz of Rice Protein
8 grams or 0.28 oz of Sesame Seeds Hulled

Protein 25g, Fat 8g, Carb 18g, Fibre 6g, 250 Kcals

Preparation

Place the nuts or seeds into the Tall Cup. Screw the Nutribullet Extractor Blade on to the top of the cup. Invert the cup, press it down into the Nutribullet Power Base and twist it into place. Blast them for 30 seconds. Put the rest of the solid ingredients into the cup and press them down below the Max Line. Add the fluid base to fill the cup up to the Max Line. Screw the Nutribullet Extractor Blade on to the top of the cup. Invert the cup, press it down into the Nutribullet Power Base and twist it into place. Blast the mixture until it is really smooth (20 or so seconds). **Enjoy!**

Mint and Pineapple Cornucopia

Ingredients

1 Cup/Handful of Red or White Cabbage (40 grams or 1½ oz)
1 Cup/Handful of Mint (40 grams or 1½ oz)
¾ Cup of Pineapple chunks (90 grams or 3 oz)
¾ Cup of sliced Cauliflower florets (90 grams or 3 oz)
200 ml / 7 fl oz of Almond Milk (Unsweetened)
25 grams or ¾ oz of Whey Protein
5 grams or 0.18 oz of Walnuts

Protein 25g, Fat 7g, Carb 18g, Fibre 10g, 250 Kcals

Preparation

Place the nuts or seeds into the Tall Cup. Screw the Nutribullet Extractor Blade on to the top of the cup. Invert the cup, press it down into the Nutribullet Power Base and twist it into place. Blast them for 30 seconds. Put the rest of the solid ingredients into the cup and press them down below the Max Line. Add the fluid base to fill the cup up to the Max Line. Screw the Nutribullet Extractor Blade on to the top of the cup. Invert the cup, press it down into the Nutribullet Power Base and twist it into place. Blast the mixture until it is really smooth (20 or so seconds). **Enjoy!**

Pineapple and Zucchini Revelation

Ingredients

1 Cup/Handful of Bok Choy (40 grams or 1½ oz)
1 Cup/Handful of Fennel (40 grams or 1½ oz)
¾ Cup of Pineapple chunks (90 grams or 3 oz)
¾ Cup of sliced Zucchini/Courgette (90 grams or 3 oz)
200 ml / 7 fl oz of Almond Milk (Unsweetened)
25 grams or ¾ oz of Whey Protein
8 grams or 0.28 oz of Walnuts

Protein 24g, Fat 9g, Carb 17g, Fibre 7g, 250 Kcals

Preparation

Place the nuts or seeds into the Tall Cup. Screw the Nutribullet Extractor Blade on to the top of the cup. Invert the cup, press it down into the Nutribullet Power Base and twist it into place. Blast them for 30 seconds. Put the rest of the solid ingredients into the cup and press them down below the Max Line. Add the fluid base to fill the cup up to the Max Line. Screw the Nutribullet Extractor Blade on to the top of the cup. Invert the cup, press it down into the Nutribullet Power Base and twist it into place. Blast the mixture until it is really smooth (20 or so seconds). **Enjoy!**

Clementine and Yellow Pepper Forever

Ingredients

2 Cups/Handfuls of Rocket/Arugura Lettuce (80 grams or 3 oz)
¾ Cup of Clementine slices (90 grams or 3 oz)
¾ Cup of sliced Yellow Pepper (90 grams or 3 oz)
200 ml / 7 fl oz of Coconut Milk
25 grams or ¾ oz of Rice Protein
8 grams or 0.28 oz of Chia Seeds

Protein 24g, Fat 5g, Carb 23g, Fibre 6g, 250 Kcals

Preparation

Place the nuts or seeds into the Tall Cup. Screw the Nutribullet Extractor Blade on to the top of the cup. Invert the cup, press it down into the Nutribullet Power Base and twist it into place. Blast them for 30 seconds. Put the rest of the solid ingredients into the cup and press them down below the Max Line. Add the fluid base to fill the cup up to the Max Line. Screw the Nutribullet Extractor Blade on to the top of the cup. Invert the cup, press it down into the Nutribullet Power Base and twist it into place. Blast the mixture until it is really smooth (20 or so seconds). **Enjoy!**

Plum Ensemble

Ingredients

1 Cup/Handful of Broccoli Florets (40 grams or 1½ oz)
1 Cup/Handful of Watercress (40 grams or 1½ oz)
¾ Cup of Plum halves (90 grams or 3 oz)
¾ Cup of diced Celeriac (90 grams or 3 oz)
200 ml / 7 fl oz of Water
25 grams or ¾ oz of Pea Protein
10 grams or 0.35 oz of Sunflower Seeds Hulled

Protein 26g, Fat 6g, Carb 22g, Fibre 5g, 250 Kcals

Preparation

Place the nuts or seeds into the Tall Cup. Screw the Nutribullet Extractor Blade on to the top of the cup. Invert the cup, press it down into the Nutribullet Power Base and twist it into place. Blast them for 30 seconds. Put the rest of the solid ingredients into the cup and press them down below the Max Line. Add the fluid base to fill the cup up to the Max Line. Screw the Nutribullet Extractor Blade on to the top of the cup. Invert the cup, press it down into the Nutribullet Power Base and twist it into place. Blast the mixture until it is really smooth (20 or so seconds). **Enjoy!**

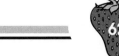

Grapefruit kisses Celery

Ingredients

2 Cups/Handfuls of Bok Choy (80 grams or 3 oz)
¾ Cup of Grapefruit segments (90 grams or 3 oz)
¾ Cup of sliced Celery (90 grams or 3 oz)
200 ml / 7 fl oz of Water
22 grams or ¾ oz of Soy Protein
17 grams or 0.60 oz of Brazil nuts

Protein 25g, Fat 12g, Carb 10g, Fibre 5g, 250 Kcals

Preparation

Place the nuts or seeds into the Tall Cup. Screw the Nutribullet Extractor Blade on to the top of the cup. Invert the cup, press it down into the Nutribullet Power Base and twist it into place. Blast them for 30 seconds. Put the rest of the solid ingredients into the cup and press them down below the Max Line. Add the fluid base to fill the cup up to the Max Line. Screw the Nutribullet Extractor Blade on to the top of the cup. Invert the cup, press it down into the Nutribullet Power Base and twist it into place. Blast the mixture until it is really smooth (20 or so seconds). **Enjoy!**

Watercress and Mint Heaven

Ingredients

1 Cup/Handful of Watercress (40 grams or 1½ oz)
1 Cup/Handful of Mint (40 grams or 1½ oz)
¾ Cup of Cherries (stoned) (90 grams or 3 oz)
¾ Cup of sliced Celery (90 grams or 3 oz)
200 ml / 7 fl oz of Hazelnut Milk
22 grams or ¾ oz of Soy Protein
3 grams or 0.11 oz of Chia Seeds

Protein 25g, Fat 5g, Carb 22g, Fibre 8g, 250 Kcals

Preparation

Place the nuts or seeds into the Tall Cup. Screw the Nutribullet Extractor Blade on to the top of the cup. Invert the cup, press it down into the Nutribullet Power Base and twist it into place. Blast them for 30 seconds. Put the rest of the solid ingredients into the cup and press them down below the Max Line. Add the fluid base to fill the cup up to the Max Line. Screw the Nutribullet Extractor Blade on to the top of the cup. Invert the cup, press it down into the Nutribullet Power Base and twist it into place. Blast the mixture until it is really smooth (20 or so seconds). **Enjoy!**

Green Cabbage partners Blueberry

Ingredients

2 Cups/Handfuls of Green Cabbage (80 grams or 3 oz)
¾ Cup of Blueberries (90 grams or 3 oz)
¾ Cup of Radishes (90 grams or 3 oz)
200 ml / 7 fl oz of Water
25 grams or ¾ oz of Rice Protein
13 grams or 0.46 oz of Cashews

Protein 25g, Fat 6g, Carb 21g, Fibre 6g, 250 Kcals

Preparation

Place the nuts or seeds into the Tall Cup. Screw the Nutribullet Extractor Blade on to the top of the cup. Invert the cup, press it down into the Nutribullet Power Base and twist it into place. Blast them for 30 seconds. Put the rest of the solid ingredients into the cup and press them down below the Max Line. Add the fluid base to fill the cup up to the Max Line. Screw the Nutribullet Extractor Blade on to the top of the cup. Invert the cup, press it down into the Nutribullet Power Base and twist it into place. Blast the mixture until it is really smooth (20 or so seconds). **Enjoy!**

Cucumber Journey

Ingredients

1 Cup/Handful of Broccoli Florets (40 grams or 1½ oz)
1 Cup/Handful of Lettuce Leaves (40 grams or 1½ oz)
¾ Cup of Water Melon chunks (90 grams or 3 oz)
¾ Cup of sliced Cucumber (90 grams or 3 oz)
200 ml / 7 fl oz of Almond Milk (Unsweetened)
25 grams or ¾ oz of Pea Protein
11 grams or 0.39 oz of Almonds

Protein 25g, Fat 9g, Carb 14g, Fibre 5g, 250 Kcals

Preparation

Place the nuts or seeds into the Tall Cup. Screw the Nutribullet Extractor Blade on to the top of the cup. Invert the cup, press it down into the Nutribullet Power Base and twist it into place. Blast them for 30 seconds. Put the rest of the solid ingredients into the cup and press them down below the Max Line. Add the fluid base to fill the cup up to the Max Line. Screw the Nutribullet Extractor Blade on to the top of the cup. Invert the cup, press it down into the Nutribullet Power Base and twist it into place. Blast the mixture until it is really smooth (20 or so seconds). **Enjoy!**

Peach and Turnip Sunset

Ingredients

1 Cup/Handful of Red or White Cabbage (40 grams or 1½ oz)
1 Cup/Handful of Bok Choy (40 grams or 1½ oz)
¾ Cup of Peach slices (90 grams or 3 oz)
¾ Cup of diced Turnip (90 grams or 3 oz)
200 ml / 7 fl oz of Water
25 grams or ¾ oz of Whey Protein
12 grams or 0.42 oz of Walnuts

Protein 24g, Fat 9g, Carb 17g, Fibre 7g, 250 Kcals

Preparation

Place the nuts or seeds into the Tall Cup. Screw the Nutribullet Extractor Blade on to the top of the cup. Invert the cup, press it down into the Nutribullet Power Base and twist it into place. Blast them for 30 seconds. Put the rest of the solid ingredients into the cup and press them down below the Max Line. Add the fluid base to fill the cup up to the Max Line. Screw the Nutribullet Extractor Blade on to the top of the cup. Invert the cup, press it down into the Nutribullet Power Base and twist it into place. Blast the mixture until it is really smooth (20 or so seconds). **Enjoy!**

Red Cabbage kisses Peach

Ingredients

1 Cup/Handful of Bok Choy (40 grams or 1½ oz)
1 Cup/Handful of Red or White Cabbage (40 grams or 1½ oz)
¾ Cup of Peach slices (90 grams or 3 oz)
¾ Cup of sliced Carrots (90 grams or 3 oz)
200 ml / 7 fl oz of Almond Milk (Unsweetened)
22 grams or ¾ oz of Soy Protein
8 grams or 0.28 oz of Hazelnuts

Protein 25g, Fat 8g, Carb 18g, Fibre 7g, 250 Kcals

Preparation

Place the nuts or seeds into the Tall Cup. Screw the Nutribullet Extractor Blade on to the top of the cup. Invert the cup, press it down into the Nutribullet Power Base and twist it into place. Blast them for 30 seconds. Put the rest of the solid ingredients into the cup and press them down below the Max Line. Add the fluid base to fill the cup up to the Max Line. Screw the Nutribullet Extractor Blade on to the top of the cup. Invert the cup, press it down into the Nutribullet Power Base and twist it into place. Blast the mixture until it is really smooth (20 or so seconds). **Enjoy!**

Mango Delivered

Ingredients

1 Cup/Handful of Rocket/Arugura Lettuce (40 grams or 1½ oz)
1 Cup/Handful of Spinach (40 grams or 1½ oz)
¾ Cup of Mango slices (90 grams or 3 oz)
¾ Cup of sliced Red Pepper (90 grams or 3 oz)
200 ml / 7 fl oz of Almond Milk (Unsweetened)
25 grams or ¾ oz of Pea Protein
4 grams or 0.14 oz of Walnuts

Protein 24g, Fat 6g, Carb 20g, Fibre 6g, 251 Kcals

Preparation

Place the nuts or seeds into the Tall Cup. Screw the Nutribullet Extractor Blade on to the top of the cup. Invert the cup, press it down into the Nutribullet Power Base and twist it into place. Blast them for 30 seconds. Put the rest of the solid ingredients into the cup and press them down below the Max Line. Add the fluid base to fill the cup up to the Max Line. Screw the Nutribullet Extractor Blade on to the top of the cup. Invert the cup, press it down into the Nutribullet Power Base and twist it into place. Blast the mixture until it is really smooth (20 or so seconds). *Enjoy!*

Fennel and Raspberry Bonanza

Ingredients

2 Cups/Handfuls of Fennel (80 grams or 3 oz)
¾ Cup of Raspberries (90 grams or 3 oz)
¾ Cup of sliced Yellow Pepper (90 grams or 3 oz)
200 ml / 7 fl oz of Water
25 grams or ¾ oz of Pea Protein
10 grams or 0.35 oz of Flax Seeds

Protein 24g, Fat 6g, Carb 15g, Fibre 12g, 251 Kcals

Preparation

Place the nuts or seeds into the Tall Cup. Screw the Nutribullet Extractor Blade on to the top of the cup. Invert the cup, press it down into the Nutribullet Power Base and twist it into place. Blast them for 30 seconds. Put the rest of the solid ingredients into the cup and press them down below the Max Line. Add the fluid base to fill the cup up to the Max Line. Screw the Nutribullet Extractor Blade on to the top of the cup. Invert the cup, press it down into the Nutribullet Power Base and twist it into place. Blast the mixture until it is really smooth (20 or so seconds). *Enjoy!*

Melon Embrace

Ingredients

1 Cup/Handful of Fennel (40 grams or 1½ oz)
1 Cup/Handful of Mint (40 grams or 1½ oz)
¾ Cup of Melon chunks (90 grams or 3 oz)
¾ Cup of sliced Celery (90 grams or 3 oz)
200 ml / 7 fl oz of Water
25 grams or ¾ oz of Pea Protein
14 grams or 0.49 oz of Sunflower Seeds Hulled

Protein 25g, Fat 8g, Carb 16g, Fibre 7g, 251 Kcals

Preparation

Place the nuts or seeds into the Tall Cup. Screw the Nutribullet Extractor Blade on to the top of the cup. Invert the cup, press it down into the Nutribullet Power Base and twist it into place. Blast them for 30 seconds. Put the rest of the solid ingredients into the cup and press them down below the Max Line. Add the fluid base to fill the cup up to the Max Line. Screw the Nutribullet Extractor Blade on to the top of the cup. Invert the cup, press it down into the Nutribullet Power Base and twist it into place. Blast the mixture until it is really smooth (20 or so seconds). **Enjoy!**

Tomato Paradise

Ingredients

1 Cup/Handful of Watercress (40 grams or 1½ oz)
1 Cup/Handful of Rocket/Arugura Lettuce (40 grams or 1½ oz)
¾ Cup of Raspberries (90 grams or 3 oz)
¾ Cup of sliced Tomato (90 grams or 3 oz)
200 ml / 7 fl oz of Hazelnut Milk
25 grams or ¾ oz of Pea Protein
3 grams or 0.11 oz of Sesame Seeds Hulled

Protein 24g, Fat 7g, Carb 17g, Fibre 8g, 251 Kcals

Preparation

Place the nuts or seeds into the Tall Cup. Screw the Nutribullet Extractor Blade on to the top of the cup. Invert the cup, press it down into the Nutribullet Power Base and twist it into place. Blast them for 30 seconds. Put the rest of the solid ingredients into the cup and press them down below the Max Line. Add the fluid base to fill the cup up to the Max Line. Screw the Nutribullet Extractor Blade on to the top of the cup. Invert the cup, press it down into the Nutribullet Power Base and twist it into place. Blast the mixture until it is really smooth (20 or so seconds). **Enjoy!**

Fig and Yellow Pepper Mist

Ingredients

1 Cup/Handful of Rocket/Arugura Lettuce (40 grams or 1½ oz)
1 Cup/Handful of Fennel (40 grams or 1½ oz)
¾ Cup of Peeled Figs (90 grams or 3 oz)
¾ Cup of sliced Yellow Pepper (90 grams or 3 oz)
200 ml / 7 fl oz of Almond Milk (Unsweetened)
25 grams or ¾ oz of Whey Protein
4 grams or 0.14 oz of Flax Seeds

Protein 23g, Fat 6g, Carb 23g, Fibre 9g, 251 Kcals

Preparation

Place the nuts or seeds into the Tall Cup. Screw the Nutribullet Extractor Blade on to the top of the cup. Invert the cup, press it down into the Nutribullet Power Base and twist it into place. Blast them for 30 seconds. Put the rest of the solid ingredients into the cup and press them down below the Max Line. Add the fluid base to fill the cup up to the Max Line. Screw the Nutribullet Extractor Blade on to the top of the cup. Invert the cup, press it down into the Nutribullet Power Base and twist it into place. Blast the mixture until it is really smooth (20 or so seconds). **Enjoy!**

Cranberry and Radish Mirage

Ingredients

1 Cup/Handful of Rocket/Arugura Lettuce (40 grams or 1½ oz)
1 Cup/Handful of Fennel (40 grams or 1½ oz)
¾ Cup of Cranberries (90 grams or 3 oz)
¾ Cup of Radishes (90 grams or 3 oz)
200 ml / 7 fl oz of Water
25 grams or ¾ oz of Whey Protein
17 grams or 0.60 oz of Chia Seeds

Protein 24g, Fat 7g, Carb 14g, Fibre 15g, 251 Kcals

Preparation

Place the nuts or seeds into the Tall Cup. Screw the Nutribullet Extractor Blade on to the top of the cup. Invert the cup, press it down into the Nutribullet Power Base and twist it into place. Blast them for 30 seconds. Put the rest of the solid ingredients into the cup and press them down below the Max Line. Add the fluid base to fill the cup up to the Max Line. Screw the Nutribullet Extractor Blade on to the top of the cup. Invert the cup, press it down into the Nutribullet Power Base and twist it into place. Blast the mixture until it is really smooth (20 or so seconds). **Enjoy!**

Fig and Red Pepper Utopia

Ingredients

1 Cup/Handful of Bok Choy (40 grams or 1½ oz)
1 Cup/Handful of Green Cabbage (40 grams or 1½ oz)
¾ Cup of Peeled Figs (90 grams or 3 oz)
¾ Cup of sliced Red Pepper (90 grams or 3 oz)
200 ml / 7 fl oz of Water
25 grams or ¾ oz of Rice Protein
7 grams or 0.25 oz of Pecans

Protein 23g, Fat 6g, Carb 23g, Fibre 7g, 251 Kcals

Preparation

Place the nuts or seeds into the Tall Cup. Screw the Nutribullet Extractor Blade on to the top of the cup. Invert the cup, press it down into the Nutribullet Power Base and twist it into place. Blast them for 30 seconds. Put the rest of the solid ingredients into the cup and press them down below the Max Line. Add the fluid base to fill the cup up to the Max Line. Screw the Nutribullet Extractor Blade on to the top of the cup. Invert the cup, press it down into the Nutribullet Power Base and twist it into place. Blast the mixture until it is really smooth (20 or so seconds). **Enjoy!**

Fennel invites Tangerine

Ingredients

1 Cup/Handful of Green Cabbage (40 grams or 1½ oz)
1 Cup/Handful of Fennel (40 grams or 1½ oz)
¾ Cup of Tangerine slices (90 grams or 3 oz)
¾ Cup of diced Swede (90 grams or 3 oz)
200 ml / 7 fl oz of Almond Milk (Unsweetened)
25 grams or ¾ oz of Rice Protein
6 grams or 0.21 oz of Sesame Seeds Hulled

Protein 24g, Fat 7g, Carb 21g, Fibre 7g, 251 Kcals

Preparation

Place the nuts or seeds into the Tall Cup. Screw the Nutribullet Extractor Blade on to the top of the cup. Invert the cup, press it down into the Nutribullet Power Base and twist it into place. Blast them for 30 seconds. Put the rest of the solid ingredients into the cup and press them down below the Max Line. Add the fluid base to fill the cup up to the Max Line. Screw the Nutribullet Extractor Blade on to the top of the cup. Invert the cup, press it down into the Nutribullet Power Base and twist it into place. Blast the mixture until it is really smooth (20 or so seconds). **Enjoy!**

Cauliflower Panacea

Ingredients

2 Cups/Handfuls of Mint (80 grams or 3 oz)
¾ Cup of Melon chunks (90 grams or 3 oz)
¾ Cup of sliced Cauliflower florets (90 grams or 3 oz)
200 ml / 7 fl oz of Water
25 grams or ¾ oz of Rice Protein
12 grams or 0.42 oz of Peanuts

Protein 28g, Fat 7g, Carb 15g, Fibre 9g, 251 Kcals

Preparation

Place the nuts or seeds into the Tall Cup. Screw the Nutribullet Extractor Blade on to the top of the cup. Invert the cup, press it down into the Nutribullet Power Base and twist it into place. Blast them for 30 seconds. Put the rest of the solid ingredients into the cup and press them down below the Max Line. Add the fluid base to fill the cup up to the Max Line. Screw the Nutribullet Extractor Blade on to the top of the cup. Invert the cup, press it down into the Nutribullet Power Base and twist it into place. Blast the mixture until it is really smooth (20 or so seconds). *Enjoy!*

Raspberry Sensation

Ingredients

1 Cup/Handful of Bok Choy (40 grams or 1½ oz)
1 Cup/Handful of Spinach (40 grams or 1½ oz)
¾ Cup of Raspberries (90 grams or 3 oz)
¾ Cup of sliced Yellow Pepper (90 grams or 3 oz)
200 ml / 7 fl oz of Hazelnut Milk
25 grams or ¾ oz of Pea Protein
1 gram or 0.04 oz of Hazelnuts

Protein 24g, Fat 6g, Carb 19g, Fibre 9g, 251 Kcals

Preparation

Place the nuts or seeds into the Tall Cup. Screw the Nutribullet Extractor Blade on to the top of the cup. Invert the cup, press it down into the Nutribullet Power Base and twist it into place. Blast them for 30 seconds. Put the rest of the solid ingredients into the cup and press them down below the Max Line. Add the fluid base to fill the cup up to the Max Line. Screw the Nutribullet Extractor Blade on to the top of the cup. Invert the cup, press it down into the Nutribullet Power Base and twist it into place. Blast the mixture until it is really smooth (20 or so seconds). *Enjoy!*

Water Melon Feast

Ingredients

1 Cup/Handful of Mint (40 grams or 1½ oz)
1 Cup/Handful of Fennel (40 grams or 1½ oz)
¾ Cup of Water Melon chunks (90 grams or 3 oz)
¾ Cup of sliced Zucchini/Courgette (90 grams or 3 oz)
200 ml / 7 fl oz of Almond Milk (Unsweetened)
25 grams or ¾ oz of Whey Protein
11 grams or 0.39 oz of Flax Seeds

Protein 25g, Fat 9g, Carb 13g, Fibre 11g, 251 Kcals

Preparation

Place the nuts or seeds into the Tall Cup. Screw the Nutribullet Extractor Blade on to the top of the cup. Invert the cup, press it down into the Nutribullet Power Base and twist it into place. Blast them for 30 seconds. Put the rest of the solid ingredients into the cup and press them down below the Max Line. Add the fluid base to fill the cup up to the Max Line. Screw the Nutribullet Extractor Blade on to the top of the cup. Invert the cup, press it down into the Nutribullet Power Base and twist it into place. Blast the mixture until it is really smooth (20 or so seconds). *Enjoy!*

Bok Choy goes Clementine

Ingredients

2 Cups/Handfuls of Bok Choy (80 grams or 3 oz)
¾ Cup of Clementine slices (90 grams or 3 oz)
¾ Cup of sliced Cauliflower florets (90 grams or 3 oz)
200 ml / 7 fl oz of Hazelnut Milk
25 grams or ¾ oz of Rice Protein
4 grams or 0.14 oz of Hazelnuts

Protein 25g, Fat 6g, Carb 22g, Fibre 5g, 251 Kcals

Preparation

Place the nuts or seeds into the Tall Cup. Screw the Nutribullet Extractor Blade on to the top of the cup. Invert the cup, press it down into the Nutribullet Power Base and twist it into place. Blast them for 30 seconds. Put the rest of the solid ingredients into the cup and press them down below the Max Line. Add the fluid base to fill the cup up to the Max Line. Screw the Nutribullet Extractor Blade on to the top of the cup. Invert the cup, press it down into the Nutribullet Power Base and twist it into place. Blast the mixture until it is really smooth (20 or so seconds). *Enjoy!*

Red Cabbage Presented

Ingredients

1 Cup/Handful of Green Cabbage (40 grams or 1½ oz)
1 Cup/Handful of Red or White Cabbage (40 grams or 1½ oz)
¾ Cup of Grapefruit segments (90 grams or 3 oz)
¾ Cup of diced Swede (90 grams or 3 oz)
200 ml / 7 fl oz of Water
25 grams or ¾ oz of Pea Protein
14 grams or 0.49 oz of Sunflower Seeds Hulled

Protein 25g, Fat 8g, Carb 19g, Fibre 5g, 251 Kcals

Preparation

Place the nuts or seeds into the Tall Cup. Screw the Nutribullet Extractor Blade on to the top of the cup. Invert the cup, press it down into the Nutribullet Power Base and twist it into place. Blast them for 30 seconds. Put the rest of the solid ingredients into the cup and press them down below the Max Line. Add the fluid base to fill the cup up to the Max Line. Screw the Nutribullet Extractor Blade on to the top of the cup. Invert the cup, press it down into the Nutribullet Power Base and twist it into place. Blast the mixture until it is really smooth (20 or so seconds). ***Enjoy!***

Swede Delight

Ingredients

2 Cups/Handfuls of Fennel (80 grams or 3 oz)
¾ Cup of Peach slices (90 grams or 3 oz)
¾ Cup of diced Swede (90 grams or 3 oz)
200 ml / 7 fl oz of Coconut Milk
25 grams or ¾ oz of Whey Protein
6 grams or 0.21 oz of Sunflower Seeds Hulled

Protein 23g, Fat 7g, Carb 23g, Fibre 8g, 251 Kcals

Preparation

Place the nuts or seeds into the Tall Cup. Screw the Nutribullet Extractor Blade on to the top of the cup. Invert the cup, press it down into the Nutribullet Power Base and twist it into place. Blast them for 30 seconds. Put the rest of the solid ingredients into the cup and press them down below the Max Line. Add the fluid base to fill the cup up to the Max Line. Screw the Nutribullet Extractor Blade on to the top of the cup. Invert the cup, press it down into the Nutribullet Power Base and twist it into place. Blast the mixture until it is really smooth (20 or so seconds). ***Enjoy!***

Orange embraces Turnip

Ingredients

2 Cups/Handfuls of Watercress (80 grams or 3 oz)
¾ Cup of Orange segments (90 grams or 3 oz)
¾ Cup of diced Turnip (90 grams or 3 oz)
200 ml / 7 fl oz of Hazelnut Milk
25 grams or ¾ oz of Pea Protein
3 grams or 0.11 oz of Sunflower Seeds Hulled

Protein 24g, Fat 6g, Carb 22g, Fibre 5g, 251 Kcals

Preparation

Place the nuts or seeds into the Tall Cup. Screw the Nutribullet Extractor Blade on to the top of the cup. Invert the cup, press it down into the Nutribullet Power Base and twist it into place. Blast them for 30 seconds. Put the rest of the solid ingredients into the cup and press them down below the Max Line. Add the fluid base to fill the cup up to the Max Line. Screw the Nutribullet Extractor Blade on to the top of the cup. Invert the cup, press it down into the Nutribullet Power Base and twist it into place. Blast the mixture until it is really smooth (20 or so seconds). **Enjoy!**

Tangerine Concerto

Ingredients

1 Cup/Handful of Mint (40 grams or 1½ oz)
1 Cup/Handful of Red or White Cabbage (40 grams or 1½ oz)
¾ Cup of Tangerine slices (90 grams or 3 oz)
¾ Cup of sliced Cucumber (90 grams or 3 oz)
200 ml / 7 fl oz of Coconut Milk
25 grams or ¾ oz of Rice Protein
5 grams or 0.18 oz of Sesame Seeds Hulled

Protein 24g, Fat 6g, Carb 22g, Fibre 6g, 251 Kcals

Preparation

Place the nuts or seeds into the Tall Cup. Screw the Nutribullet Extractor Blade on to the top of the cup. Invert the cup, press it down into the Nutribullet Power Base and twist it into place. Blast them for 30 seconds. Put the rest of the solid ingredients into the cup and press them down below the Max Line. Add the fluid base to fill the cup up to the Max Line. Screw the Nutribullet Extractor Blade on to the top of the cup. Invert the cup, press it down into the Nutribullet Power Base and twist it into place. Blast the mixture until it is really smooth (20 or so seconds). **Enjoy!**

Red Cabbage in Pear

Ingredients

2 Cups/Handfuls of Red or White Cabbage (80 grams or 3 oz)
¾ Cup of Pear slices (90 grams or 3 oz)
¾ Cup of sliced Fine Beans (90 grams or 3 oz)
200 ml / 7 fl oz of Coconut Milk
25 grams or ¾ oz of Pea Protein
2 grams or 0.07 oz of Peanuts

Protein 23g, Fat 4g, Carb 27g, Fibre 7g, 251 Kcals

Preparation

Place the nuts or seeds into the Tall Cup. Screw the Nutribullet Extractor Blade on to the top of the cup. Invert the cup, press it down into the Nutribullet Power Base and twist it into place. Blast them for 30 seconds. Put the rest of the solid ingredients into the cup and press them down below the Max Line. Add the fluid base to fill the cup up to the Max Line. Screw the Nutribullet Extractor Blade on to the top of the cup. Invert the cup, press it down into the Nutribullet Power Base and twist it into place. Blast the mixture until it is really smooth (20 or so seconds). **Enjoy!**

Broccoli and Kiwi Potion

Ingredients

2 Cups/Handfuls of Broccoli Florets (80 grams or 3 oz)
¾ Cup of Kiwi Fruit slices (90 grams or 3 oz)
¾ Cup of Radishes (90 grams or 3 oz)
200 ml / 7 fl oz of Water
25 grams or ¾ oz of Pea Protein
11 grams or 0.39 oz of Chia Seeds

Protein 25g, Fat 5g, Carb 19g, Fibre 10g, 251 Kcals

Preparation

Place the nuts or seeds into the Tall Cup. Screw the Nutribullet Extractor Blade on to the top of the cup. Invert the cup, press it down into the Nutribullet Power Base and twist it into place. Blast them for 30 seconds. Put the rest of the solid ingredients into the cup and press them down below the Max Line. Add the fluid base to fill the cup up to the Max Line. Screw the Nutribullet Extractor Blade on to the top of the cup. Invert the cup, press it down into the Nutribullet Power Base and twist it into place. Blast the mixture until it is really smooth (20 or so seconds). **Enjoy!**

Fig and Tomato Wonder

Ingredients

1 Cup/Handful of Fennel (40 grams or 1½ oz)
1 Cup/Handful of Bok Choy (40 grams or 1½ oz)
¾ Cup of Peeled Figs (90 grams or 3 oz)
¾ Cup of sliced Tomato (90 grams or 3 oz)
200 ml / 7 fl oz of Almond Milk (Unsweetened)
25 grams or ¾ oz of Pea Protein
4 grams or 0.14 oz of Almonds

Protein 24g, Fat 6g, Carb 22g, Fibre 7g, 251 Kcals

Preparation

Place the nuts or seeds into the Tall Cup. Screw the Nutribullet Extractor Blade on to the top of the cup. Invert the cup, press it down into the Nutribullet Power Base and twist it into place. Blast them for 30 seconds. Put the rest of the solid ingredients into the cup and press them down below the Max Line. Add the fluid base to fill the cup up to the Max Line. Screw the Nutribullet Extractor Blade on to the top of the cup. Invert the cup, press it down into the Nutribullet Power Base and twist it into place. Blast the mixture until it is really smooth (20 or so seconds). **Enjoy!**

Cranberry partners Fine Bean

Ingredients

1 Cup/Handful of Broccoli Florets (40 grams or 1½ oz)
1 Cup/Handful of Mint (40 grams or 1½ oz)
¾ Cup of Cranberries (90 grams or 3 oz)
¾ Cup of sliced Fine Beans (90 grams or 3 oz)
200 ml / 7 fl oz of Water
25 grams or ¾ oz of Whey Protein
11 grams or 0.39 oz of Pumpkin Seeds

Protein 26g, Fat 7g, Carb 15g, Fibre 12g, 251 Kcals

Preparation

Place the nuts or seeds into the Tall Cup. Screw the Nutribullet Extractor Blade on to the top of the cup. Invert the cup, press it down into the Nutribullet Power Base and twist it into place. Blast them for 30 seconds. Put the rest of the solid ingredients into the cup and press them down below the Max Line. Add the fluid base to fill the cup up to the Max Line. Screw the Nutribullet Extractor Blade on to the top of the cup. Invert the cup, press it down into the Nutribullet Power Base and twist it into place. Blast the mixture until it is really smooth (20 or so seconds). **Enjoy!**

Pear and Beetroot Invigorator

Ingredients

1 Cup/Handful of Red or White Cabbage (40 grams or 1½ oz)
1 Cup/Handful of Lettuce Leaves (40 grams or 1½ oz)
¾ Cup of Pear slices (90 grams or 3 oz)
¾ Cup of diced Beetroot (90 grams or 3 oz)
200 ml / 7 fl oz of Water
25 grams or ¾ oz of Whey Protein
9 grams or 0.32 oz of Flax Seeds

Protein 23g, Fat 5g, Carb 23g, Fibre 11g, 251 Kcals

Preparation

Place the nuts or seeds into the Tall Cup. Screw the Nutribullet Extractor Blade on to the top of the cup. Invert the cup, press it down into the Nutribullet Power Base and twist it into place. Blast them for 30 seconds. Put the rest of the solid ingredients into the cup and press them down below the Max Line. Add the fluid base to fill the cup up to the Max Line. Screw the Nutribullet Extractor Blade on to the top of the cup. Invert the cup, press it down into the Nutribullet Power Base and twist it into place. Blast the mixture until it is really smooth (20 or so seconds). ***Enjoy!***

Mango kisses Zucchini

Ingredients

1 Cup/Handful of Broccoli Florets (40 grams or 1½ oz)
1 Cup/Handful of Mint (40 grams or 1½ oz)
¾ Cup of Mango slices (90 grams or 3 oz)
¾ Cup of sliced Zucchini/Courgette (90 grams or 3 oz)
200 ml / 7 fl oz of Almond Milk (Unsweetened)
25 grams or ¾ oz of Rice Protein
6 grams or 0.21 oz of Flax Seeds

Protein 26g, Fat 6g, Carb 19g, Fibre 9g, 251 Kcals

Preparation

Place the nuts or seeds into the Tall Cup. Screw the Nutribullet Extractor Blade on to the top of the cup. Invert the cup, press it down into the Nutribullet Power Base and twist it into place. Blast them for 30 seconds. Put the rest of the solid ingredients into the cup and press them down below the Max Line. Add the fluid base to fill the cup up to the Max Line. Screw the Nutribullet Extractor Blade on to the top of the cup. Invert the cup, press it down into the Nutribullet Power Base and twist it into place. Blast the mixture until it is really smooth (20 or so seconds). ***Enjoy!***

Bok Choy befriends Lettuce

Ingredients

1 Cup/Handful of Bok Choy (40 grams or 1½ oz)
1 Cup/Handful of Lettuce Leaves (40 grams or 1½ oz)
¾ Cup of Apricot halves (90 grams or 3 oz)
¾ Cup of sliced Carrots (90 grams or 3 oz)
200 ml / 7 fl oz of Coconut Milk
22 grams or ¾ oz of Soy Protein
5 grams or 0.18 oz of Pecans

Protein 24g, Fat 6g, Carb 22g, Fibre 6g, 251 Kcals

Preparation

Place the nuts or seeds into the Tall Cup. Screw the Nutribullet Extractor Blade on to the top of the cup. Invert the cup, press it down into the Nutribullet Power Base and twist it into place. Blast them for 30 seconds. Put the rest of the solid ingredients into the cup and press them down below the Max Line. Add the fluid base to fill the cup up to the Max Line. Screw the Nutribullet Extractor Blade on to the top of the cup. Invert the cup, press it down into the Nutribullet Power Base and twist it into place. Blast the mixture until it is really smooth (20 or so seconds). **Enjoy!**

Watercress in Papaya

Ingredients

2 Cups/Handfuls of Watercress (80 grams or 3 oz)
¾ Cup of Papaya (90 grams or 3 oz)
¾ Cup of diced Swede (90 grams or 3 oz)
200 ml / 7 fl oz of Water
25 grams or ¾ oz of Rice Protein
13 grams or 0.46 oz of Walnuts

Protein 25g, Fat 9g, Carb 17g, Fibre 5g, 251 Kcals

Preparation

Place the nuts or seeds into the Tall Cup. Screw the Nutribullet Extractor Blade on to the top of the cup. Invert the cup, press it down into the Nutribullet Power Base and twist it into place. Blast them for 30 seconds. Put the rest of the solid ingredients into the cup and press them down below the Max Line. Add the fluid base to fill the cup up to the Max Line. Screw the Nutribullet Extractor Blade on to the top of the cup. Invert the cup, press it down into the Nutribullet Power Base and twist it into place. Blast the mixture until it is really smooth (20 or so seconds). **Enjoy!**

Grapefruit and Radish Infusion

Ingredients

2 Cups/Handfuls of Red or White Cabbage (80 grams or 3 oz)
¾ Cup of Grapefruit segments (90 grams or 3 oz)
¾ Cup of Radishes (90 grams or 3 oz)
200 ml / 7 fl oz of Hazelnut Milk
25 grams or ¾ oz of Whey Protein
5 grams or 0.18 oz of Hazelnuts

Protein 23g, Fat 8g, Carb 20g, Fibre 7g, 251 Kcals

Preparation

Place the nuts or seeds into the Tall Cup. Screw the Nutribullet Extractor Blade on to the top of the cup. Invert the cup, press it down into the Nutribullet Power Base and twist it into place. Blast them for 30 seconds. Put the rest of the solid ingredients into the cup and press them down below the Max Line. Add the fluid base to fill the cup up to the Max Line. Screw the Nutribullet Extractor Blade on to the top of the cup. Invert the cup, press it down into the Nutribullet Power Base and twist it into place. Blast the mixture until it is really smooth (20 or so seconds). *Enjoy!*

Melon and Tomato Waistline

Ingredients

1 Cup/Handful of Watercress (40 grams or 1½ oz)
1 Cup/Handful of Mint (40 grams or 1½ oz)
¾ Cup of Melon chunks (90 grams or 3 oz)
¾ Cup of sliced Tomato (90 grams or 3 oz)
200 ml / 7 fl oz of Coconut Milk
25 grams or ¾ oz of Rice Protein
9 grams or 0.32 oz of Flax Seeds

Protein 25g, Fat 6g, Carb 19g, Fibre 7g, 251 Kcals

Preparation

Place the nuts or seeds into the Tall Cup. Screw the Nutribullet Extractor Blade on to the top of the cup. Invert the cup, press it down into the Nutribullet Power Base and twist it into place. Blast them for 30 seconds. Put the rest of the solid ingredients into the cup and press them down below the Max Line. Add the fluid base to fill the cup up to the Max Line. Screw the Nutribullet Extractor Blade on to the top of the cup. Invert the cup, press it down into the Nutribullet Power Base and twist it into place. Blast the mixture until it is really smooth (20 or so seconds). *Enjoy!*

Mint and Kiwi Kiss

Ingredients

1 Cup/Handful of Green Cabbage (40 grams or 1½ oz)
1 Cup/Handful of Mint (40 grams or 1½ oz)
¾ Cup of Kiwi Fruit slices (90 grams or 3 oz)
¾ Cup of Radishes (90 grams or 3 oz)
200 ml / 7 fl oz of Coconut Milk
22 grams or ¾ oz of Soy Protein
5 grams or 0.18 oz of Sesame Seeds Hulled

Protein 24g, Fat 6g, Carb 21g, Fibre 8g, 251 Kcals

Preparation

Place the nuts or seeds into the Tall Cup. Screw the Nutribullet Extractor Blade on to the top of the cup. Invert the cup, press it down into the Nutribullet Power Base and twist it into place. Blast them for 30 seconds. Put the rest of the solid ingredients into the cup and press them down below the Max Line. Add the fluid base to fill the cup up to the Max Line. Screw the Nutribullet Extractor Blade on to the top of the cup. Invert the cup, press it down into the Nutribullet Power Base and twist it into place. Blast the mixture until it is really smooth (20 or so seconds). **Enjoy!**

Green Cabbage Contradiction

Ingredients

1 Cup/Handful of Red or White Cabbage (40 grams or 1½ oz)
1 Cup/Handful of Green Cabbage (40 grams or 1½ oz)
¾ Cup of Papaya (90 grams or 3 oz)
¾ Cup of diced Turnip (90 grams or 3 oz)
200 ml / 7 fl oz of Hazelnut Milk
25 grams or ¾ oz of Pea Protein
1 gram or 0.04 oz of Sesame Seeds Hulled

Protein 23g, Fat 5g, Carb 25g, Fibre 6g, 252 Kcals

Preparation

Place the nuts or seeds into the Tall Cup. Screw the Nutribullet Extractor Blade on to the top of the cup. Invert the cup, press it down into the Nutribullet Power Base and twist it into place. Blast them for 30 seconds. Put the rest of the solid ingredients into the cup and press them down below the Max Line. Add the fluid base to fill the cup up to the Max Line. Screw the Nutribullet Extractor Blade on to the top of the cup. Invert the cup, press it down into the Nutribullet Power Base and twist it into place. Blast the mixture until it is really smooth (20 or so seconds). **Enjoy!**

Apricot meets Carrot

Ingredients

1 Cup/Handful of Watercress (40 grams or 1½ oz)
1 Cup/Handful of Spinach (40 grams or 1½ oz)
¾ Cup of Apricot halves (90 grams or 3 oz)
¾ Cup of sliced Carrots (90 grams or 3 oz)
200 ml / 7 fl oz of Coconut Milk
25 grams or ¾ oz of Pea Protein
3 grams or 0.11 oz of Cashews

Protein 24g, Fat 5g, Carb 24g, Fibre 5g, 252 Kcals

Preparation

Place the nuts or seeds into the Tall Cup. Screw the Nutribullet Extractor Blade on to the top of the cup. Invert the cup, press it down into the Nutribullet Power Base and twist it into place. Blast them for 30 seconds. Put the rest of the solid ingredients into the cup and press them down below the Max Line. Add the fluid base to fill the cup up to the Max Line. Screw the Nutribullet Extractor Blade on to the top of the cup. Invert the cup, press it down into the Nutribullet Power Base and twist it into place. Blast the mixture until it is really smooth (20 or so seconds). *Enjoy!*

Green Cabbage and Apple Salad

Ingredients

2 Cups/Handfuls of Green Cabbage (80 grams or 3 oz)
¾ Cup of Apple slices (90 grams or 3 oz)
¾ Cup of sliced Cauliflower florets (90 grams or 3 oz)
200 ml / 7 fl oz of Coconut Milk
25 grams or ¾ oz of Rice Protein
5 grams or 0.18 oz of Almonds

Protein 24g, Fat 5g, Carb 24g, Fibre 6g, 252 Kcals

Preparation

Place the nuts or seeds into the Tall Cup. Screw the Nutribullet Extractor Blade on to the top of the cup. Invert the cup, press it down into the Nutribullet Power Base and twist it into place. Blast them for 30 seconds. Put the rest of the solid ingredients into the cup and press them down below the Max Line. Add the fluid base to fill the cup up to the Max Line. Screw the Nutribullet Extractor Blade on to the top of the cup. Invert the cup, press it down into the Nutribullet Power Base and twist it into place. Blast the mixture until it is really smooth (20 or so seconds). *Enjoy!*

Green Cabbage and Peach Nectar

Ingredients

1 Cup/Handful of Green Cabbage (40 grams or 1½ oz)
1 Cup/Handful of Bok Choy (40 grams or 1½ oz)
¾ Cup of Peach slices (90 grams or 3 oz)
¾ Cup of sliced Red Pepper (90 grams or 3 oz)
200 ml / 7 fl oz of Hazelnut Milk
25 grams or ¾ oz of Whey Protein
4 grams or 0.14 oz of Flax Seeds

Protein 23g, Fat 7g, Carb 21g, Fibre 8g, 252 Kcals

Preparation

Place the nuts or seeds into the Tall Cup. Screw the Nutribullet Extractor Blade on to the top of the cup. Invert the cup, press it down into the Nutribullet Power Base and twist it into place. Blast them for 30 seconds. Put the rest of the solid ingredients into the cup and press them down below the Max Line. Add the fluid base to fill the cup up to the Max Line. Screw the Nutribullet Extractor Blade on to the top of the cup. Invert the cup, press it down into the Nutribullet Power Base and twist it into place. Blast the mixture until it is really smooth (20 or so seconds). **Enjoy!**

Pineapple joins Turnip

Ingredients

2 Cups/Handfuls of Spinach (80 grams or 3 oz)
¾ Cup of Pineapple chunks (90 grams or 3 oz)
¾ Cup of diced Turnip (90 grams or 3 oz)
200 ml / 7 fl oz of Almond Milk (Unsweetened)
25 grams or ¾ oz of Rice Protein
8 grams or 0.28 oz of Cashews

Protein 26g, Fat 6g, Carb 21g, Fibre 6g, 252 Kcals

Preparation

Place the nuts or seeds into the Tall Cup. Screw the Nutribullet Extractor Blade on to the top of the cup. Invert the cup, press it down into the Nutribullet Power Base and twist it into place. Blast them for 30 seconds. Put the rest of the solid ingredients into the cup and press them down below the Max Line. Add the fluid base to fill the cup up to the Max Line. Screw the Nutribullet Extractor Blade on to the top of the cup. Invert the cup, press it down into the Nutribullet Power Base and twist it into place. Blast the mixture until it is really smooth (20 or so seconds). **Enjoy!**

Fig Garden

Ingredients

1 Cup/Handful of Red or White Cabbage (40 grams or 1½ oz)
1 Cup/Handful of Spinach (40 grams or 1½ oz)
¾ Cup of Peeled Figs (90 grams or 3 oz)
¾ Cup of sliced Cauliflower florets (90 grams or 3 oz)
200 ml / 7 fl oz of Water
25 grams or ¾ oz of Pea Protein
7 grams or 0.25 oz of Peanuts

Protein 25g, Fat 5g, Carb 23g, Fibre 7g, 252 Kcals

Preparation

Place the nuts or seeds into the Tall Cup. Screw the Nutribullet Extractor Blade on to the top of the cup. Invert the cup, press it down into the Nutribullet Power Base and twist it into place. Blast them for 30 seconds. Put the rest of the solid ingredients into the cup and press them down below the Max Line. Add the fluid base to fill the cup up to the Max Line. Screw the Nutribullet Extractor Blade on to the top of the cup. Invert the cup, press it down into the Nutribullet Power Base and twist it into place. Blast the mixture until it is really smooth (20 or so seconds). **Enjoy!**

Melon meets Turnip

Ingredients

1 Cup/Handful of Green Cabbage (40 grams or 1½ oz)
1 Cup/Handful of Spinach (40 grams or 1½ oz)
¾ Cup of Melon chunks (90 grams or 3 oz)
¾ Cup of diced Turnip (90 grams or 3 oz)
200 ml / 7 fl oz of Coconut Milk
22 grams or ¾ oz of Soy Protein
8 grams or 0.28 oz of Hazelnuts

Protein 24g, Fat 7g, Carb 21g, Fibre 5g, 252 Kcals

Preparation

Place the nuts or seeds into the Tall Cup. Screw the Nutribullet Extractor Blade on to the top of the cup. Invert the cup, press it down into the Nutribullet Power Base and twist it into place. Blast them for 30 seconds. Put the rest of the solid ingredients into the cup and press them down below the Max Line. Add the fluid base to fill the cup up to the Max Line. Screw the Nutribullet Extractor Blade on to the top of the cup. Invert the cup, press it down into the Nutribullet Power Base and twist it into place. Blast the mixture until it is really smooth (20 or so seconds). **Enjoy!**

Kiwi in Green Pepper

Ingredients

1 Cup/Handful of Fennel (40 grams or 1½ oz)
1 Cup/Handful of Rocket/Arugura Lettuce (40 grams or 1½ oz)
¾ Cup of Kiwi Fruit slices (90 grams or 3 oz)
¾ Cup of sliced Green Pepper (90 grams or 3 oz)
200 ml / 7 fl oz of Coconut Milk
25 grams or ¾ oz of Rice Protein
4 grams or 0.14 oz of Pecans

Protein 23g, Fat 6g, Carb 24g, Fibre 6g, 252 Kcals

Preparation

Place the nuts or seeds into the Tall Cup. Screw the Nutribullet Extractor Blade on to the top of the cup. Invert the cup, press it down into the Nutribullet Power Base and twist it into place. Blast them for 30 seconds. Put the rest of the solid ingredients into the cup and press them down below the Max Line. Add the fluid base to fill the cup up to the Max Line. Screw the Nutribullet Extractor Blade on to the top of the cup. Invert the cup, press it down into the Nutribullet Power Base and twist it into place. Blast the mixture until it is really smooth (20 or so seconds). **Enjoy!**

Fig invites Red Pepper

Ingredients

2 Cups/Handfuls of Broccoli Florets (80 grams or 3 oz)
¾ Cup of Peeled Figs (90 grams or 3 oz)
¾ Cup of sliced Red Pepper (90 grams or 3 oz)
200 ml / 7 fl oz of Water
22 grams or ¾ oz of Soy Protein
8 grams or 0.28 oz of Peanuts

Protein 26g, Fat 5g, Carb 23g, Fibre 7g, 252 Kcals

Preparation

Place the nuts or seeds into the Tall Cup. Screw the Nutribullet Extractor Blade on to the top of the cup. Invert the cup, press it down into the Nutribullet Power Base and twist it into place. Blast them for 30 seconds. Put the rest of the solid ingredients into the cup and press them down below the Max Line. Add the fluid base to fill the cup up to the Max Line. Screw the Nutribullet Extractor Blade on to the top of the cup. Invert the cup, press it down into the Nutribullet Power Base and twist it into place. Blast the mixture until it is really smooth (20 or so seconds). **Enjoy!**

Spinach and Cranberry Potion

Ingredients

1 Cup/Handful of Fennel (40 grams or 1½ oz)
1 Cup/Handful of Spinach (40 grams or 1½ oz)
¾ Cup of Cranberries (90 grams or 3 oz)
¾ Cup of diced Celeriac (90 grams or 3 oz)
200 ml / 7 fl oz of Coconut Milk
22 grams or ¾ oz of Soy Protein
4 grams or 0.14 oz of Brazil nuts

Protein 24g, Fat 5g, Carb 22g, Fibre 8g, 252 Kcals

Preparation

Place the nuts or seeds into the Tall Cup. Screw the Nutribullet Extractor Blade on to the top of the cup. Invert the cup, press it down into the Nutribullet Power Base and twist it into place. Blast them for 30 seconds. Put the rest of the solid ingredients into the cup and press them down below the Max Line. Add the fluid base to fill the cup up to the Max Line. Screw the Nutribullet Extractor Blade on to the top of the cup. Invert the cup, press it down into the Nutribullet Power Base and twist it into place. Blast the mixture until it is really smooth (20 or so seconds). **Enjoy!**

Bok Choy Elixir

Ingredients

1 Cup/Handful of Bok Choy (40 grams or 1½ oz)
1 Cup/Handful of Red or White Cabbage (40 grams or 1½ oz)
¾ Cup of Banana slices (90 grams or 3 oz)
¾ Cup of sliced Yellow Pepper (90 grams or 3 oz)
200 ml / 7 fl oz of Almond Milk (Unsweetened)
25 grams or ¾ oz of Rice Protein
2 grams or 0.07 oz of Cashews

Protein 24g, Fat 4g, Carb 28g, Fibre 5g, 252 Kcals

Preparation

Place the nuts or seeds into the Tall Cup. Screw the Nutribullet Extractor Blade on to the top of the cup. Invert the cup, press it down into the Nutribullet Power Base and twist it into place. Blast them for 30 seconds. Put the rest of the solid ingredients into the cup and press them down below the Max Line. Add the fluid base to fill the cup up to the Max Line. Screw the Nutribullet Extractor Blade on to the top of the cup. Invert the cup, press it down into the Nutribullet Power Base and twist it into place. Blast the mixture until it is really smooth (20 or so seconds). **Enjoy!**

Watercress Heaven

Ingredients

1 Cup/Handful of Watercress (40 grams or 1½ oz)
1 Cup/Handful of Rocket/Arugura Lettuce (40 grams or 1½ oz)
¾ Cup of Orange segments (90 grams or 3 oz)
¾ Cup of diced Celeriac (90 grams or 3 oz)
200 ml / 7 fl oz of Water
22 grams or ¾ oz of Soy Protein
13 grams or 0.46 oz of Almonds

Protein 26g, Fat 7g, Carb 18g, Fibre 6g, 252 Kcals

Preparation

Place the nuts or seeds into the Tall Cup. Screw the Nutribullet Extractor Blade on to the top of the cup. Invert the cup, press it down into the Nutribullet Power Base and twist it into place. Blast them for 30 seconds. Put the rest of the solid ingredients into the cup and press them down below the Max Line. Add the fluid base to fill the cup up to the Max Line. Screw the Nutribullet Extractor Blade on to the top of the cup. Invert the cup, press it down into the Nutribullet Power Base and twist it into place. Blast the mixture until it is really smooth (20 or so seconds). **Enjoy!**

Spinach goes Mango

Ingredients

1 Cup/Handful of Spinach (40 grams or 1½ oz)
1 Cup/Handful of Lettuce Leaves (40 grams or 1½ oz)
¾ Cup of Mango slices (90 grams or 3 oz)
¾ Cup of sliced Yellow Pepper (90 grams or 3 oz)
200 ml / 7 fl oz of Coconut Milk
22 grams or ¾ oz of Soy Protein
5 grams or 0.18 oz of Brazil nuts

Protein 24g, Fat 6g, Carb 24g, Fibre 4g, 252 Kcals

Preparation

Place the nuts or seeds into the Tall Cup. Screw the Nutribullet Extractor Blade on to the top of the cup. Invert the cup, press it down into the Nutribullet Power Base and twist it into place. Blast them for 30 seconds. Put the rest of the solid ingredients into the cup and press them down below the Max Line. Add the fluid base to fill the cup up to the Max Line. Screw the Nutribullet Extractor Blade on to the top of the cup. Invert the cup, press it down into the Nutribullet Power Base and twist it into place. Blast the mixture until it is really smooth (20 or so seconds). **Enjoy!**

Mint and Green Cabbage Blossom

Ingredients

1 Cup/Handful of Mint (40 grams or 1½ oz)
1 Cup/Handful of Green Cabbage (40 grams or 1½ oz)
¾ Cup of Raspberries (90 grams or 3 oz)
¾ Cup of sliced Celery (90 grams or 3 oz)
200 ml / 7 fl oz of Water
25 grams or ¾ oz of Whey Protein
10 grams or 0.35 oz of Pecans

Protein 23g, Fat 9g, Carb 10g, Fibre 14g, 252 Kcals

Preparation

Place the nuts or seeds into the Tall Cup. Screw the Nutribullet Extractor Blade on to the top of the cup. Invert the cup, press it down into the Nutribullet Power Base and twist it into place. Blast them for 30 seconds. Put the rest of the solid ingredients into the cup and press them down below the Max Line. Add the fluid base to fill the cup up to the Max Line. Screw the Nutribullet Extractor Blade on to the top of the cup. Invert the cup, press it down into the Nutribullet Power Base and twist it into place. Blast the mixture until it is really smooth (20 or so seconds). **Enjoy!**

Watercress and Fennel Fiesta

Ingredients

1 Cup/Handful of Watercress (40 grams or 1½ oz)
1 Cup/Handful of Fennel (40 grams or 1½ oz)
¾ Cup of Mango slices (90 grams or 3 oz)
¾ Cup of sliced Tomato (90 grams or 3 oz)
200 ml / 7 fl oz of Hazelnut Milk
25 grams or ¾ oz of Pea Protein
1 gram or 0.04 oz of Pumpkin Seeds

Protein 23g, Fat 5g, Carb 25g, Fibre 5g, 252 Kcals

Preparation

Place the nuts or seeds into the Tall Cup. Screw the Nutribullet Extractor Blade on to the top of the cup. Invert the cup, press it down into the Nutribullet Power Base and twist it into place. Blast them for 30 seconds. Put the rest of the solid ingredients into the cup and press them down below the Max Line. Add the fluid base to fill the cup up to the Max Line. Screw the Nutribullet Extractor Blade on to the top of the cup. Invert the cup, press it down into the Nutribullet Power Base and twist it into place. Blast the mixture until it is really smooth (20 or so seconds). **Enjoy!**

Water Melon and Yellow Pepper Dance

Ingredients

1 Cup/Handful of Red or White Cabbage (40 grams or 1½ oz)
1 Cup/Handful of Fennel (40 grams or 1½ oz)
¾ Cup of Water Melon chunks (90 grams or 3 oz)
¾ Cup of sliced Yellow Pepper (90 grams or 3 oz)
200 ml / 7 fl oz of Hazelnut Milk
22 grams or ¾ oz of Soy Protein
6 grams or 0.21 oz of Cashews

Protein 24g, Fat 6g, Carb 23g, Fibre 4g, 252 Kcals

Preparation

Place the nuts or seeds into the Tall Cup. Screw the Nutribullet Extractor Blade on to the top of the cup. Invert the cup, press it down into the Nutribullet Power Base and twist it into place. Blast them for 30 seconds. Put the rest of the solid ingredients into the cup and press them down below the Max Line. Add the fluid base to fill the cup up to the Max Line. Screw the Nutribullet Extractor Blade on to the top of the cup. Invert the cup, press it down into the Nutribullet Power Base and twist it into place. Blast the mixture until it is really smooth (20 or so seconds). **Enjoy!**

Broccoli and Plum Detente

Ingredients

2 Cups/Handfuls of Broccoli Florets (80 grams or 3 oz)
¾ Cup of Plum halves (90 grams or 3 oz)
¾ Cup of sliced Tomato (90 grams or 3 oz)
200 ml / 7 fl oz of Water
25 grams or ¾ oz of Pea Protein
10 grams or 0.35 oz of Brazil nuts

Protein 25g, Fat 8g, Carb 18g, Fibre 5g, 252 Kcals

Preparation

Place the nuts or seeds into the Tall Cup. Screw the Nutribullet Extractor Blade on to the top of the cup. Invert the cup, press it down into the Nutribullet Power Base and twist it into place. Blast them for 30 seconds. Put the rest of the solid ingredients into the cup and press them down below the Max Line. Add the fluid base to fill the cup up to the Max Line. Screw the Nutribullet Extractor Blade on to the top of the cup. Invert the cup, press it down into the Nutribullet Power Base and twist it into place. Blast the mixture until it is really smooth (20 or so seconds). **Enjoy!**

Water Melon and Swede Seduction

Ingredients

1 Cup/Handful of Rocket/Arugura Lettuce (40 grams or 1½ oz)
1 Cup/Handful of Green Cabbage (40 grams or 1½ oz)
¾ Cup of Water Melon chunks (90 grams or 3 oz)
¾ Cup of diced Swede (90 grams or 3 oz)
200 ml / 7 fl oz of Hazelnut Milk
25 grams or ¾ oz of Pea Protein
4 grams or 0.14 oz of Almonds

Protein 23g, Fat 7g, Carb 22g, Fibre 5g, 252 Kcals

Preparation

Place the nuts or seeds into the Tall Cup. Screw the Nutribullet Extractor Blade on to the top of the cup. Invert the cup, press it down into the Nutribullet Power Base and twist it into place. Blast them for 30 seconds. Put the rest of the solid ingredients into the cup and press them down below the Max Line. Add the fluid base to fill the cup up to the Max Line. Screw the Nutribullet Extractor Blade on to the top of the cup. Invert the cup, press it down into the Nutribullet Power Base and twist it into place. Blast the mixture until it is really smooth (20 or so seconds). **Enjoy!**

Pear Surprise

Ingredients

2 Cups/Handfuls of Red or White Cabbage (80 grams or 3 oz)
¾ Cup of Pear slices (90 grams or 3 oz)
¾ Cup of Radishes (90 grams or 3 oz)
200 ml / 7 fl oz of Almond Milk (Unsweetened)
25 grams or ¾ oz of Whey Protein
6 grams or 0.21 oz of Pecans

Protein 22g, Fat 8g, Carb 20g, Fibre 9g, 252 Kcals

Preparation

Place the nuts or seeds into the Tall Cup. Screw the Nutribullet Extractor Blade on to the top of the cup. Invert the cup, press it down into the Nutribullet Power Base and twist it into place. Blast them for 30 seconds. Put the rest of the solid ingredients into the cup and press them down below the Max Line. Add the fluid base to fill the cup up to the Max Line. Screw the Nutribullet Extractor Blade on to the top of the cup. Invert the cup, press it down into the Nutribullet Power Base and twist it into place. Blast the mixture until it is really smooth (20 or so seconds). **Enjoy!**

Mint Debut

Ingredients

1 Cup/Handful of Red or White Cabbage (40 grams or 1½ oz)
1 Cup/Handful of Mint (40 grams or 1½ oz)
¾ Cup of Plum halves (90 grams or 3 oz)
¾ Cup of sliced Cucumber (90 grams or 3 oz)
200 ml / 7 fl oz of Coconut Milk
22 grams or ¾ oz of Soy Protein
8 grams or 0.28 oz of Pumpkin Seeds

Protein 25g, Fat 6g, Carb 20g, Fibre 6g, 252 Kcals

Preparation

Place the nuts or seeds into the Tall Cup. Screw the Nutribullet Extractor Blade on to the top of the cup. Invert the cup, press it down into the Nutribullet Power Base and twist it into place. Blast them for 30 seconds. Put the rest of the solid ingredients into the cup and press them down below the Max Line. Add the fluid base to fill the cup up to the Max Line. Screw the Nutribullet Extractor Blade on to the top of the cup. Invert the cup, press it down into the Nutribullet Power Base and twist it into place. Blast the mixture until it is really smooth (20 or so seconds). **Enjoy!**

Fennel kisses Spinach

Ingredients

1 Cup/Handful of Fennel (40 grams or 1½ oz)
1 Cup/Handful of Spinach (40 grams or 1½ oz)
¾ Cup of Peeled Figs (90 grams or 3 oz)
¾ Cup of sliced Red Pepper (90 grams or 3 oz)
200 ml / 7 fl oz of Coconut Milk
22 grams or ¾ oz of Soy Protein
2 grams or 0.07 oz of Peanuts

Protein 24g, Fat 4g, Carb 27g, Fibre 7g, 252 Kcals

Preparation

Place the nuts or seeds into the Tall Cup. Screw the Nutribullet Extractor Blade on to the top of the cup. Invert the cup, press it down into the Nutribullet Power Base and twist it into place. Blast them for 30 seconds. Put the rest of the solid ingredients into the cup and press them down below the Max Line. Add the fluid base to fill the cup up to the Max Line. Screw the Nutribullet Extractor Blade on to the top of the cup. Invert the cup, press it down into the Nutribullet Power Base and twist it into place. Blast the mixture until it is really smooth (20 or so seconds). **Enjoy!**

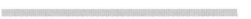

Peach Orchard

Ingredients

1 Cup/Handful of Mint (40 grams or 1½ oz)
1 Cup/Handful of Red or White Cabbage (40 grams or 1½ oz)
¾ Cup of Peach slices (90 grams or 3 oz)
¾ Cup of diced Beetroot (90 grams or 3 oz)
200 ml / 7 fl oz of Coconut Milk
25 grams or ¾ oz of Rice Protein
3 grams or 0.11 oz of Sunflower Seeds Hulled

Protein 25g, Fat 4g, Carb 24g, Fibre 8g, 252 Kcals

Preparation

Place the nuts or seeds into the Tall Cup. Screw the Nutribullet Extractor Blade on to the top of the cup. Invert the cup, press it down into the Nutribullet Power Base and twist it into place. Blast them for 30 seconds. Put the rest of the solid ingredients into the cup and press them down below the Max Line. Add the fluid base to fill the cup up to the Max Line. Screw the Nutribullet Extractor Blade on to the top of the cup. Invert the cup, press it down into the Nutribullet Power Base and twist it into place. Blast the mixture until it is really smooth (20 or so seconds). **Enjoy!**

Mint and Water Melon Waterfall

Ingredients

1 Cup/Handful of Fennel (40 grams or 1½ oz)
1 Cup/Handful of Mint (40 grams or 1½ oz)
¾ Cup of Water Melon chunks (90 grams or 3 oz)
¾ Cup of Radishes (90 grams or 3 oz)
200 ml / 7 fl oz of Almond Milk (Unsweetened)
25 grams or ¾ oz of Pea Protein
11 grams or 0.39 oz of Chia Seeds

Protein 25g, Fat 7g, Carb 14g, Fibre 10g, 252 Kcals

Preparation

Place the nuts or seeds into the Tall Cup. Screw the Nutribullet Extractor Blade on to the top of the cup. Invert the cup, press it down into the Nutribullet Power Base and twist it into place. Blast them for 30 seconds. Put the rest of the solid ingredients into the cup and press them down below the Max Line. Add the fluid base to fill the cup up to the Max Line. Screw the Nutribullet Extractor Blade on to the top of the cup. Invert the cup, press it down into the Nutribullet Power Base and twist it into place. Blast the mixture until it is really smooth (20 or so seconds). **Enjoy!**

Bok Choy joins Apricot

Ingredients

2 Cups/Handfuls of Bok Choy (80 grams or 3 oz)
¾ Cup of Apricot halves (90 grams or 3 oz)
¾ Cup of sliced Carrots (90 grams or 3 oz)
200 ml / 7 fl oz of Coconut Milk
25 grams or ¾ oz of Whey Protein
5 grams or 0.18 oz of Cashews

Protein 23g, Fat 6g, Carb 24g, Fibre 7g, 252 Kcals

Preparation

Place the nuts or seeds into the Tall Cup. Screw the Nutribullet Extractor Blade on to the top of the cup. Invert the cup, press it down into the Nutribullet Power Base and twist it into place. Blast them for 30 seconds. Put the rest of the solid ingredients into the cup and press them down below the Max Line. Add the fluid base to fill the cup up to the Max Line. Screw the Nutribullet Extractor Blade on to the top of the cup. Invert the cup, press it down into the Nutribullet Power Base and twist it into place. Blast the mixture until it is really smooth (20 or so seconds). **Enjoy!**

Broccoli and Cranberry Medley

Ingredients

1 Cup/Handful of Green Cabbage (40 grams or 1½ oz)
1 Cup/Handful of Broccoli Florets (40 grams or 1½ oz)
¾ Cup of Cranberries (90 grams or 3 oz)
¾ Cup of sliced Red Pepper (90 grams or 3 oz)
200 ml / 7 fl oz of Almond Milk (Unsweetened)
25 grams or ¾ oz of Pea Protein
6 grams or 0.21 oz of Flax Seeds

Protein 24g, Fat 6g, Carb 16g, Fibre 11g, 252 Kcals

Preparation

Place the nuts or seeds into the Tall Cup. Screw the Nutribullet Extractor Blade on to the top of the cup. Invert the cup, press it down into the Nutribullet Power Base and twist it into place. Blast them for 30 seconds. Put the rest of the solid ingredients into the cup and press them down below the Max Line. Add the fluid base to fill the cup up to the Max Line. Screw the Nutribullet Extractor Blade on to the top of the cup. Invert the cup, press it down into the Nutribullet Power Base and twist it into place. Blast the mixture until it is really smooth (20 or so seconds). **Enjoy!**

Lettuce and Strawberry Soother

Ingredients

1 Cup/Handful of Lettuce Leaves (40 grams or 1½ oz)
1 Cup/Handful of Bok Choy (40 grams or 1½ oz)
¾ Cup of Strawberries (90 grams or 3 oz)
¾ Cup of sliced Red Pepper (90 grams or 3 oz)
200 ml / 7 fl oz of Water
22 grams or ¾ oz of Soy Protein
15 grams or 0.53 oz of Brazil nuts

Protein 25g, Fat 11g, Carb 11g, Fibre 6g, 252 Kcals

Preparation

Place the nuts or seeds into the Tall Cup. Screw the Nutribullet Extractor Blade on to the top of the cup. Invert the cup, press it down into the Nutribullet Power Base and twist it into place. Blast them for 30 seconds. Put the rest of the solid ingredients into the cup and press them down below the Max Line. Add the fluid base to fill the cup up to the Max Line. Screw the Nutribullet Extractor Blade on to the top of the cup. Invert the cup, press it down into the Nutribullet Power Base and twist it into place. Blast the mixture until it is really smooth (20 or so seconds). *Enjoy!*

Raspberry joins Cucumber

Ingredients

1 Cup/Handful of Rocket/Arugura Lettuce (40 grams or 1½ oz)
1 Cup/Handful of Mint (40 grams or 1½ oz)
¾ Cup of Raspberries (90 grams or 3 oz)
¾ Cup of sliced Cucumber (90 grams or 3 oz)
200 ml / 7 fl oz of Almond Milk (Unsweetened)
25 grams or ¾ oz of Whey Protein
9 grams or 0.32 oz of Peanuts

Protein 26g, Fat 9g, Carb 10g, Fibre 13g, 252 Kcals

Preparation

Place the nuts or seeds into the Tall Cup. Screw the Nutribullet Extractor Blade on to the top of the cup. Invert the cup, press it down into the Nutribullet Power Base and twist it into place. Blast them for 30 seconds. Put the rest of the solid ingredients into the cup and press them down below the Max Line. Add the fluid base to fill the cup up to the Max Line. Screw the Nutribullet Extractor Blade on to the top of the cup. Invert the cup, press it down into the Nutribullet Power Base and twist it into place. Blast the mixture until it is really smooth (20 or so seconds). *Enjoy!*

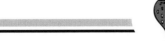

Rocket hugs Peach

Ingredients

1 Cup/Handful of Green Cabbage (40 grams or 1½ oz)
1 Cup/Handful of Rocket/Arugura Lettuce (40 grams or 1½ oz)
¾ Cup of Peach slices (90 grams or 3 oz)
¾ Cup of sliced Fine Beans (90 grams or 3 oz)
200 ml / 7 fl oz of Water
25 grams or ¾ oz of Pea Protein
14 grams or 0.49 oz of Cashews

Protein 26g, Fat 8g, Carb 19g, Fibre 5g, 252 Kcals

Preparation

Place the nuts or seeds into the Tall Cup. Screw the Nutribullet Extractor Blade on to the top of the cup. Invert the cup, press it down into the Nutribullet Power Base and twist it into place. Blast them for 30 seconds. Put the rest of the solid ingredients into the cup and press them down below the Max Line. Add the fluid base to fill the cup up to the Max Line. Screw the Nutribullet Extractor Blade on to the top of the cup. Invert the cup, press it down into the Nutribullet Power Base and twist it into place. Blast the mixture until it is really smooth (20 or so seconds). **Enjoy!**

Red Grape Refrain

Ingredients

1 Cup/Handful of Broccoli Florets (40 grams or 1½ oz)
1 Cup/Handful of Rocket/Arugura Lettuce (40 grams or 1½ oz)
¾ Cup of Red Grapes (90 grams or 3 oz)
¾ Cup of sliced Green Pepper (90 grams or 3 oz)
200 ml / 7 fl oz of Almond Milk (Unsweetened)
25 grams or ¾ oz of Rice Protein
6 grams or 0.21 oz of Pumpkin Seeds

Protein 25g, Fat 6g, Carb 24g, Fibre 5g, 252 Kcals

Preparation

Place the nuts or seeds into the Tall Cup. Screw the Nutribullet Extractor Blade on to the top of the cup. Invert the cup, press it down into the Nutribullet Power Base and twist it into place. Blast them for 30 seconds. Put the rest of the solid ingredients into the cup and press them down below the Max Line. Add the fluid base to fill the cup up to the Max Line. Screw the Nutribullet Extractor Blade on to the top of the cup. Invert the cup, press it down into the Nutribullet Power Base and twist it into place. Blast the mixture until it is really smooth (20 or so seconds). **Enjoy!**

Rocket invites Melon

Ingredients

1 Cup/Handful of Rocket/Arugura Lettuce (40 grams or 1½ oz)
1 Cup/Handful of Bok Choy (40 grams or 1½ oz)
¾ Cup of Melon chunks (90 grams or 3 oz)
¾ Cup of diced Swede (90 grams or 3 oz)
200 ml / 7 fl oz of Coconut Milk
25 grams or ¾ oz of Pea Protein
6 grams or 0.21 oz of Pecans

Protein 23g, Fat 7g, Carb 21g, Fibre 4g, 252 Kcals

Preparation

Place the nuts or seeds into the Tall Cup. Screw the Nutribullet Extractor Blade on to the top of the cup. Invert the cup, press it down into the Nutribullet Power Base and twist it into place. Blast them for 30 seconds. Put the rest of the solid ingredients into the cup and press them down below the Max Line. Add the fluid base to fill the cup up to the Max Line. Screw the Nutribullet Extractor Blade on to the top of the cup. Invert the cup, press it down into the Nutribullet Power Base and twist it into place. Blast the mixture until it is really smooth (20 or so seconds). **Enjoy!**

Carrot Symphony

Ingredients

1 Cup/Handful of Spinach (40 grams or 1½ oz)
1 Cup/Handful of Watercress (40 grams or 1½ oz)
¾ Cup of Guava (90 grams or 3 oz)
¾ Cup of sliced Carrots (90 grams or 3 oz)
200 ml / 7 fl oz of Almond Milk (Unsweetened)
25 grams or ¾ oz of Whey Protein
3 grams or 0.11 oz of Pecans

Protein 25g, Fat 7g, Carb 17g, Fibre 11g, 252 Kcals

Preparation

Place the nuts or seeds into the Tall Cup. Screw the Nutribullet Extractor Blade on to the top of the cup. Invert the cup, press it down into the Nutribullet Power Base and twist it into place. Blast them for 30 seconds. Put the rest of the solid ingredients into the cup and press them down below the Max Line. Add the fluid base to fill the cup up to the Max Line. Screw the Nutribullet Extractor Blade on to the top of the cup. Invert the cup, press it down into the Nutribullet Power Base and twist it into place. Blast the mixture until it is really smooth (20 or so seconds). **Enjoy!**

Radish Twist

Ingredients

1 Cup/Handful of Watercress (40 grams or 1½ oz)
1 Cup/Handful of Rocket/Arugura Lettuce (40 grams or 1½ oz)
¾ Cup of Tangerine slices (90 grams or 3 oz)
¾ Cup of Radishes (90 grams or 3 oz)
200 ml / 7 fl oz of Coconut Milk
22 grams or ¾ oz of Soy Protein
10 grams or 0.35 oz of Cashews

Protein 25g, Fat 7g, Carb 22g, Fibre 4g, 252 Kcals

Preparation

Place the nuts or seeds into the Tall Cup. Screw the Nutribullet Extractor Blade on to the top of the cup. Invert the cup, press it down into the Nutribullet Power Base and twist it into place. Blast them for 30 seconds. Put the rest of the solid ingredients into the cup and press them down below the Max Line. Add the fluid base to fill the cup up to the Max Line. Screw the Nutribullet Extractor Blade on to the top of the cup. Invert the cup, press it down into the Nutribullet Power Base and twist it into place. Blast the mixture until it is really smooth (20 or so seconds). **Enjoy!**

Bok Choy meets Raspberry

Ingredients

1 Cup/Handful of Bok Choy (40 grams or 1½ oz)
1 Cup/Handful of Red or White Cabbage (40 grams or 1½ oz)
¾ Cup of Raspberries (90 grams or 3 oz)
¾ Cup of diced Swede (90 grams or 3 oz)
200 ml / 7 fl oz of Coconut Milk
25 grams or ¾ oz of Pea Protein
3 grams or 0.11 oz of Pecans

Protein 23g, Fat 6g, Carb 20g, Fibre 9g, 252 Kcals

Preparation

Place the nuts or seeds into the Tall Cup. Screw the Nutribullet Extractor Blade on to the top of the cup. Invert the cup, press it down into the Nutribullet Power Base and twist it into place. Blast them for 30 seconds. Put the rest of the solid ingredients into the cup and press them down below the Max Line. Add the fluid base to fill the cup up to the Max Line. Screw the Nutribullet Extractor Blade on to the top of the cup. Invert the cup, press it down into the Nutribullet Power Base and twist it into place. Blast the mixture until it is really smooth (20 or so seconds). **Enjoy!**

Spinach and Raspberry Royale

Ingredients

1 Cup/Handful of Bok Choy (40 grams or 1½ oz)
1 Cup/Handful of Spinach (40 grams or 1½ oz)
¾ Cup of Raspberries (90 grams or 3 oz)
¾ Cup of sliced Cucumber (90 grams or 3 oz)
200 ml / 7 fl oz of Hazelnut Milk
25 grams or ¾ oz of Pea Protein
4 grams or 0.14 oz of Flax Seeds

Protein 24g, Fat 7g, Carb 16g, Fibre 9g, 253 Kcals

Preparation

Place the nuts or seeds into the Tall Cup. Screw the Nutribullet Extractor Blade on to the top of the cup. Invert the cup, press it down into the Nutribullet Power Base and twist it into place. Blast them for 30 seconds. Put the rest of the solid ingredients into the cup and press them down below the Max Line. Add the fluid base to fill the cup up to the Max Line. Screw the Nutribullet Extractor Blade on to the top of the cup. Invert the cup, press it down into the Nutribullet Power Base and twist it into place. Blast the mixture until it is really smooth (20 or so seconds). *Enjoy!*

Apricot and Swede Revision

Ingredients

2 Cups/Handfuls of Mint (80 grams or 3 oz)
¾ Cup of Apricot halves (90 grams or 3 oz)
¾ Cup of diced Swede (90 grams or 3 oz)
200 ml / 7 fl oz of Coconut Milk
25 grams or ¾ oz of Pea Protein
1 gram or 0.04 oz of Pecans

Protein 24g, Fat 4g, Carb 22g, Fibre 9g, 253 Kcals

Preparation

Place the nuts or seeds into the Tall Cup. Screw the Nutribullet Extractor Blade on to the top of the cup. Invert the cup, press it down into the Nutribullet Power Base and twist it into place. Blast them for 30 seconds. Put the rest of the solid ingredients into the cup and press them down below the Max Line. Add the fluid base to fill the cup up to the Max Line. Screw the Nutribullet Extractor Blade on to the top of the cup. Invert the cup, press it down into the Nutribullet Power Base and twist it into place. Blast the mixture until it is really smooth (20 or so seconds). *Enjoy!*

Blueberry Utopia

Ingredients

1 Cup/Handful of Bok Choy (40 grams or 1½ oz)
1 Cup/Handful of Green Cabbage (40 grams or 1½ oz)
¾ Cup of Blueberries (90 grams or 3 oz)
¾ Cup of sliced Cucumber (90 grams or 3 oz)
200 ml / 7 fl oz of Water
25 grams or ¾ oz of Rice Protein
17 grams or 0.60 oz of Chia Seeds

Protein 25g, Fat 6g, Carb 18g, Fibre 10g, 253 Kcals

Preparation

Place the nuts or seeds into the Tall Cup. Screw the Nutribullet Extractor Blade on to the top of the cup. Invert the cup, press it down into the Nutribullet Power Base and twist it into place. Blast them for 30 seconds. Put the rest of the solid ingredients into the cup and press them down below the Max Line. Add the fluid base to fill the cup up to the Max Line. Screw the Nutribullet Extractor Blade on to the top of the cup. Invert the cup, press it down into the Nutribullet Power Base and twist it into place. Blast the mixture until it is really smooth (20 or so seconds). **Enjoy!**

Kiwi Sonata

Ingredients

1 Cup/Handful of Lettuce Leaves (40 grams or 1½ oz)
1 Cup/Handful of Watercress (40 grams or 1½ oz)
¾ Cup of Kiwi Fruit slices (90 grams or 3 oz)
¾ Cup of sliced Fine Beans (90 grams or 3 oz)
200 ml / 7 fl oz of Almond Milk (Unsweetened)
25 grams or ¾ oz of Rice Protein
8 grams or 0.28 oz of Peanuts

Protein 27g, Fat 7g, Carb 17g, Fibre 7g, 253 Kcals

Preparation

Place the nuts or seeds into the Tall Cup. Screw the Nutribullet Extractor Blade on to the top of the cup. Invert the cup, press it down into the Nutribullet Power Base and twist it into place. Blast them for 30 seconds. Put the rest of the solid ingredients into the cup and press them down below the Max Line. Add the fluid base to fill the cup up to the Max Line. Screw the Nutribullet Extractor Blade on to the top of the cup. Invert the cup, press it down into the Nutribullet Power Base and twist it into place. Blast the mixture until it is really smooth (20 or so seconds). **Enjoy!**

Fennel Extravaganza

Ingredients

1 Cup/Handful of Fennel (40 grams or 1½ oz)
1 Cup/Handful of Mint (40 grams or 1½ oz)
¾ Cup of Blackberries (90 grams or 3 oz)
¾ Cup of sliced Green Pepper (90 grams or 3 oz)
200 ml / 7 fl oz of Coconut Milk
22 grams or ¾ oz of Soy Protein
6 grams or 0.21 oz of Pecans

Protein 24g, Fat 7g, Carb 16g, Fibre 11g, 253 Kcals

Preparation

Place the nuts or seeds into the Tall Cup. Screw the Nutribullet Extractor Blade on to the top of the cup. Invert the cup, press it down into the Nutribullet Power Base and twist it into place. Blast them for 30 seconds. Put the rest of the solid ingredients into the cup and press them down below the Max Line. Add the fluid base to fill the cup up to the Max Line. Screw the Nutribullet Extractor Blade on to the top of the cup. Invert the cup, press it down into the Nutribullet Power Base and twist it into place. Blast the mixture until it is really smooth (20 or so seconds). **Enjoy!**

Kiwi and Celeriac Booster

Ingredients

1 Cup/Handful of Broccoli Florets (40 grams or 1½ oz)
1 Cup/Handful of Spinach (40 grams or 1½ oz)
¾ Cup of Kiwi Fruit slices (90 grams or 3 oz)
¾ Cup of diced Celeriac (90 grams or 3 oz)
200 ml / 7 fl oz of Water
22 grams or ¾ oz of Soy Protein
8 grams or 0.28 oz of Brazil nuts

Protein 26g, Fat 6g, Carb 21g, Fibre 7g, 253 Kcals

Preparation

Place the nuts or seeds into the Tall Cup. Screw the Nutribullet Extractor Blade on to the top of the cup. Invert the cup, press it down into the Nutribullet Power Base and twist it into place. Blast them for 30 seconds. Put the rest of the solid ingredients into the cup and press them down below the Max Line. Add the fluid base to fill the cup up to the Max Line. Screw the Nutribullet Extractor Blade on to the top of the cup. Invert the cup, press it down into the Nutribullet Power Base and twist it into place. Blast the mixture until it is really smooth (20 or so seconds). **Enjoy!**

Nectarine and Beetroot Opera

Ingredients

2 Cups/Handfuls of Bok Choy (80 grams or 3 oz)
¾ Cup of Nectarine segments (90 grams or 3 oz)
¾ Cup of diced Beetroot (90 grams or 3 oz)
200 ml / 7 fl oz of Coconut Milk
22 grams or ¾ oz of Soy Protein
7 grams or 0.25 oz of Pumpkin Seeds

Protein 25g, Fat 6g, Carb 22g, Fibre 5g, 253 Kcals

Preparation

Place the nuts or seeds into the Tall Cup. Screw the Nutribullet Extractor Blade on to the top of the cup. Invert the cup, press it down into the Nutribullet Power Base and twist it into place. Blast them for 30 seconds. Put the rest of the solid ingredients into the cup and press them down below the Max Line. Add the fluid base to fill the cup up to the Max Line. Screw the Nutribullet Extractor Blade on to the top of the cup. Invert the cup, press it down into the Nutribullet Power Base and twist it into place. Blast the mixture until it is really smooth (20 or so seconds). **Enjoy!**

Broccoli Cocktail

Ingredients

1 Cup/Handful of Broccoli Florets (40 grams or 1½ oz)
1 Cup/Handful of Green Cabbage (40 grams or 1½ oz)
¾ Cup of Water Melon chunks (90 grams or 3 oz)
¾ Cup of sliced Cauliflower florets (90 grams or 3 oz)
200 ml / 7 fl oz of Almond Milk (Unsweetened)
25 grams or ¾ oz of Whey Protein
10 grams or 0.35 oz of Sesame Seeds Hulled

Protein 26g, Fat 10g, Carb 14g, Fibre 8g, 253 Kcals

Preparation

Place the nuts or seeds into the Tall Cup. Screw the Nutribullet Extractor Blade on to the top of the cup. Invert the cup, press it down into the Nutribullet Power Base and twist it into place. Blast them for 30 seconds. Put the rest of the solid ingredients into the cup and press them down below the Max Line. Add the fluid base to fill the cup up to the Max Line. Screw the Nutribullet Extractor Blade on to the top of the cup. Invert the cup, press it down into the Nutribullet Power Base and twist it into place. Blast the mixture until it is really smooth (20 or so seconds). **Enjoy!**

Red Cabbage and Orange Fix

Ingredients

1 Cup/Handful of Mint (40 grams or 1½ oz)
1 Cup/Handful of Red or White Cabbage (40 grams or 1½ oz)
¾ Cup of Orange segments (90 grams or 3 oz)
¾ Cup of sliced Carrots (90 grams or 3 oz)
200 ml / 7 fl oz of Coconut Milk
25 grams or ¾ oz of Whey Protein
2 grams or 0.07 oz of Chia Seeds

Protein 23g, Fat 4g, Carb 25g, Fibre 11g, 253 Kcals

Preparation

Place the nuts or seeds into the Tall Cup. Screw the Nutribullet Extractor Blade on to the top of the cup. Invert the cup, press it down into the Nutribullet Power Base and twist it into place. Blast them for 30 seconds. Put the rest of the solid ingredients into the cup and press them down below the Max Line. Add the fluid base to fill the cup up to the Max Line. Screw the Nutribullet Extractor Blade on to the top of the cup. Invert the cup, press it down into the Nutribullet Power Base and twist it into place. Blast the mixture until it is really smooth (20 or so seconds). **Enjoy!**

Red Cabbage and Peach Sunrise

Ingredients

1 Cup/Handful of Spinach (40 grams or 1½ oz)
1 Cup/Handful of Red or White Cabbage (40 grams or 1½ oz)
¾ Cup of Peach slices (90 grams or 3 oz)
¾ Cup of Radishes (90 grams or 3 oz)
200 ml / 7 fl oz of Coconut Milk
25 grams or ¾ oz of Whey Protein
8 grams or 0.28 oz of Sesame Seeds Hulled

Protein 24g, Fat 8g, Carb 19g, Fibre 7g, 253 Kcals

Preparation

Place the nuts or seeds into the Tall Cup. Screw the Nutribullet Extractor Blade on to the top of the cup. Invert the cup, press it down into the Nutribullet Power Base and twist it into place. Blast them for 30 seconds. Put the rest of the solid ingredients into the cup and press them down below the Max Line. Add the fluid base to fill the cup up to the Max Line. Screw the Nutribullet Extractor Blade on to the top of the cup. Invert the cup, press it down into the Nutribullet Power Base and twist it into place. Blast the mixture until it is really smooth (20 or so seconds). **Enjoy!**

Celery Blend

Ingredients

1 Cup/Handful of Red or White Cabbage (40 grams or 1½ oz)
1 Cup/Handful of Green Cabbage (40 grams or 1½ oz)
¾ Cup of Papaya (90 grams or 3 oz)
¾ Cup of sliced Celery (90 grams or 3 oz)
200 ml / 7 fl oz of Almond Milk (Unsweetened)
25 grams or ¾ oz of Rice Protein
9 grams or 0.32 oz of Walnuts

Protein 24g, Fat 9g, Carb 16g, Fibre 6g, 253 Kcals

Preparation

Place the nuts or seeds into the Tall Cup. Screw the Nutribullet Extractor Blade on to the top of the cup. Invert the cup, press it down into the Nutribullet Power Base and twist it into place. Blast them for 30 seconds. Put the rest of the solid ingredients into the cup and press them down below the Max Line. Add the fluid base to fill the cup up to the Max Line. Screw the Nutribullet Extractor Blade on to the top of the cup. Invert the cup, press it down into the Nutribullet Power Base and twist it into place. Blast the mixture until it is really smooth (20 or so seconds). **Enjoy!**

Lettuce and Bok Choy Consortium

Ingredients

1 Cup/Handful of Lettuce Leaves (40 grams or 1½ oz)
1 Cup/Handful of Bok Choy (40 grams or 1½ oz)
¾ Cup of Clementine slices (90 grams or 3 oz)
¾ Cup of sliced Zucchini/Courgette (90 grams or 3 oz)
200 ml / 7 fl oz of Almond Milk (Unsweetened)
25 grams or ¾ oz of Pea Protein
10 grams or 0.35 oz of Pumpkin Seeds

Protein 26g, Fat 8g, Carb 16g, Fibre 5g, 253 Kcals

Preparation

Place the nuts or seeds into the Tall Cup. Screw the Nutribullet Extractor Blade on to the top of the cup. Invert the cup, press it down into the Nutribullet Power Base and twist it into place. Blast them for 30 seconds. Put the rest of the solid ingredients into the cup and press them down below the Max Line. Add the fluid base to fill the cup up to the Max Line. Screw the Nutribullet Extractor Blade on to the top of the cup. Invert the cup, press it down into the Nutribullet Power Base and twist it into place. Blast the mixture until it is really smooth (20 or so seconds). **Enjoy!**

Green Pepper Fix

Ingredients

2 Cups/Handfuls of Mint (80 grams or 3 oz)
¾ Cup of Mango slices (90 grams or 3 oz)
¾ Cup of sliced Green Pepper (90 grams or 3 oz)
200 ml / 7 fl oz of Water
25 grams or ¾ oz of Rice Protein
11 grams or 0.39 oz of Chia Seeds

Protein 26g, Fat 5g, Carb 19g, Fibre 12g, 253 Kcals

Preparation

Place the nuts or seeds into the Tall Cup. Screw the Nutribullet Extractor Blade on to the top of the cup. Invert the cup, press it down into the Nutribullet Power Base and twist it into place. Blast them for 30 seconds. Put the rest of the solid ingredients into the cup and press them down below the Max Line. Add the fluid base to fill the cup up to the Max Line. Screw the Nutribullet Extractor Blade on to the top of the cup. Invert the cup, press it down into the Nutribullet Power Base and twist it into place. Blast the mixture until it is really smooth (20 or so seconds). *Enjoy!*

Watercress and Bok Choy Galaxy

Ingredients

1 Cup/Handful of Watercress (40 grams or 1½ oz)
1 Cup/Handful of Bok Choy (40 grams or 1½ oz)
¾ Cup of Red Grapes (90 grams or 3 oz)
¾ Cup of sliced Celery (90 grams or 3 oz)
200 ml / 7 fl oz of Hazelnut Milk
25 grams or ¾ oz of Rice Protein
3 grams or 0.11 oz of Cashews

Protein 24g, Fat 5g, Carb 27g, Fibre 4g, 253 Kcals

Preparation

Place the nuts or seeds into the Tall Cup. Screw the Nutribullet Extractor Blade on to the top of the cup. Invert the cup, press it down into the Nutribullet Power Base and twist it into place. Blast them for 30 seconds. Put the rest of the solid ingredients into the cup and press them down below the Max Line. Add the fluid base to fill the cup up to the Max Line. Screw the Nutribullet Extractor Blade on to the top of the cup. Invert the cup, press it down into the Nutribullet Power Base and twist it into place. Blast the mixture until it is really smooth (20 or so seconds). *Enjoy!*

Lettuce and Apple Creation

Ingredients

1 Cup/Handful of Lettuce Leaves (40 grams or 1½ oz)
1 Cup/Handful of Broccoli Florets (40 grams or 1½ oz)
¾ Cup of Apple slices (90 grams or 3 oz)
¾ Cup of diced Turnip (90 grams or 3 oz)
200 ml / 7 fl oz of Water
25 grams or ¾ oz of Pea Protein
10 grams or 0.35 oz of Sesame Seeds Hulled

Protein 24g, Fat 7g, Carb 19g, Fibre 6g, 253 Kcals

Preparation

Place the nuts or seeds into the Tall Cup. Screw the Nutribullet Extractor Blade on to the top of the cup. Invert the cup, press it down into the Nutribullet Power Base and twist it into place. Blast them for 30 seconds. Put the rest of the solid ingredients into the cup and press them down below the Max Line. Add the fluid base to fill the cup up to the Max Line. Screw the Nutribullet Extractor Blade on to the top of the cup. Invert the cup, press it down into the Nutribullet Power Base and twist it into place. Blast the mixture until it is really smooth (20 or so seconds). **Enjoy!**

Spinach and Apricot Treat

Ingredients

1 Cup/Handful of Bok Choy (40 grams or 1½ oz)
1 Cup/Handful of Spinach (40 grams or 1½ oz)
¾ Cup of Apricot halves (90 grams or 3 oz)
¾ Cup of sliced Green Pepper (90 grams or 3 oz)
200 ml / 7 fl oz of Coconut Milk
25 grams or ¾ oz of Whey Protein
7 grams or 0.25 oz of Hazelnuts

Protein 24g, Fat 8g, Carb 20g, Fibre 7g, 254 Kcals

Preparation

Place the nuts or seeds into the Tall Cup. Screw the Nutribullet Extractor Blade on to the top of the cup. Invert the cup, press it down into the Nutribullet Power Base and twist it into place. Blast them for 30 seconds. Put the rest of the solid ingredients into the cup and press them down below the Max Line. Add the fluid base to fill the cup up to the Max Line. Screw the Nutribullet Extractor Blade on to the top of the cup. Invert the cup, press it down into the Nutribullet Power Base and twist it into place. Blast the mixture until it is really smooth (20 or so seconds). **Enjoy!**

Lettuce and Watercress Extravaganza

Ingredients

1 Cup/Handful of Lettuce Leaves (40 grams or 1½ oz)
1 Cup/Handful of Watercress (40 grams or 1½ oz)
¾ Cup of Water Melon chunks (90 grams or 3 oz)
¾ Cup of diced Celeriac (90 grams or 3 oz)
200 ml / 7 fl oz of Almond Milk (Unsweetened)
25 grams or ¾ oz of Rice Protein
9 grams or 0.32 oz of Walnuts

Protein 25g, Fat 9g, Carb 17g, Fibre 4g, 254 Kcals

Preparation

Place the nuts or seeds into the Tall Cup. Screw the Nutribullet Extractor Blade on to the top of the cup. Invert the cup, press it down into the Nutribullet Power Base and twist it into place. Blast them for 30 seconds. Put the rest of the solid ingredients into the cup and press them down below the Max Line. Add the fluid base to fill the cup up to the Max Line. Screw the Nutribullet Extractor Blade on to the top of the cup. Invert the cup, press it down into the Nutribullet Power Base and twist it into place. Blast the mixture until it is really smooth (20 or so seconds). **Enjoy!**

Nectarine Bliss

Ingredients

1 Cup/Handful of Bok Choy (40 grams or 1½ oz)
1 Cup/Handful of Spinach (40 grams or 1½ oz)
¾ Cup of Nectarine segments (90 grams or 3 oz)
¾ Cup of sliced Cauliflower florets (90 grams or 3 oz)
200 ml / 7 fl oz of Hazelnut Milk
25 grams or ¾ oz of Whey Protein
4 grams or 0.14 oz of Hazelnuts

Protein 25g, Fat 8g, Carb 20g, Fibre 7g, 254 Kcals

Preparation

Place the nuts or seeds into the Tall Cup. Screw the Nutribullet Extractor Blade on to the top of the cup. Invert the cup, press it down into the Nutribullet Power Base and twist it into place. Blast them for 30 seconds. Put the rest of the solid ingredients into the cup and press them down below the Max Line. Add the fluid base to fill the cup up to the Max Line. Screw the Nutribullet Extractor Blade on to the top of the cup. Invert the cup, press it down into the Nutribullet Power Base and twist it into place. Blast the mixture until it is really smooth (20 or so seconds). **Enjoy!**

Mango and Cucumber Cornucopia

Ingredients

1 Cup/Handful of Spinach (40 grams or 1½ oz)
1 Cup/Handful of Bok Choy (40 grams or 1½ oz)
¾ Cup of Mango slices (90 grams or 3 oz)
¾ Cup of sliced Cucumber (90 grams or 3 oz)
200 ml / 7 fl oz of Coconut Milk
25 grams or ¾ oz of Pea Protein
6 grams or 0.21 oz of Cashews

Protein 24g, Fat 6g, Carb 24g, Fibre 4g, 254 Kcals

Preparation

Place the nuts or seeds into the Tall Cup. Screw the Nutribullet Extractor Blade on to the top of the cup. Invert the cup, press it down into the Nutribullet Power Base and twist it into place. Blast them for 30 seconds. Put the rest of the solid ingredients into the cup and press them down below the Max Line. Add the fluid base to fill the cup up to the Max Line. Screw the Nutribullet Extractor Blade on to the top of the cup. Invert the cup, press it down into the Nutribullet Power Base and twist it into place. Blast the mixture until it is really smooth (20 or so seconds). **Enjoy!**

Mint partners Red Cabbage

Ingredients

1 Cup/Handful of Mint (40 grams or 1½ oz)
1 Cup/Handful of Red or White Cabbage (40 grams or 1½ oz)
¾ Cup of Orange segments (90 grams or 3 oz)
¾ Cup of diced Turnip (90 grams or 3 oz)
200 ml / 7 fl oz of Almond Milk (Unsweetened)
25 grams or ¾ oz of Rice Protein
7 grams or 0.25 oz of Flax Seeds

Protein 26g, Fat 6g, Carb 18g, Fibre 10g, 254 Kcals

Preparation

Place the nuts or seeds into the Tall Cup. Screw the Nutribullet Extractor Blade on to the top of the cup. Invert the cup, press it down into the Nutribullet Power Base and twist it into place. Blast them for 30 seconds. Put the rest of the solid ingredients into the cup and press them down below the Max Line. Add the fluid base to fill the cup up to the Max Line. Screw the Nutribullet Extractor Blade on to the top of the cup. Invert the cup, press it down into the Nutribullet Power Base and twist it into place. Blast the mixture until it is really smooth (20 or so seconds). **Enjoy!**

Watercress in Red Cabbage

Ingredients

1 Cup/Handful of Watercress (40 grams or 1½ oz)
1 Cup/Handful of Red or White Cabbage (40 grams or 1½ oz)
¾ Cup of Guava (90 grams or 3 oz)
¾ Cup of diced Beetroot (90 grams or 3 oz)
200 ml / 7 fl oz of Water
25 grams or ¾ oz of Rice Protein
8 grams or 0.28 oz of Cashews

Protein 27g, Fat 5g, Carb 21g, Fibre 9g, 254 Kcals

Preparation

Place the nuts or seeds into the Tall Cup. Screw the Nutribullet Extractor Blade on to the top of the cup. Invert the cup, press it down into the Nutribullet Power Base and twist it into place. Blast them for 30 seconds. Put the rest of the solid ingredients into the cup and press them down below the Max Line. Add the fluid base to fill the cup up to the Max Line. Screw the Nutribullet Extractor Blade on to the top of the cup. Invert the cup, press it down into the Nutribullet Power Base and twist it into place. Blast the mixture until it is really smooth (20 or so seconds). **Enjoy!**

Rocket Extracted

Ingredients

1 Cup/Handful of Red or White Cabbage (40 grams or 1½ oz)
1 Cup/Handful of Rocket/Arugura Lettuce (40 grams or 1½ oz)
¾ Cup of Cherries (stoned) (90 grams or 3 oz)
¾ Cup of sliced Red Pepper (90 grams or 3 oz)
200 ml / 7 fl oz of Water
25 grams or ¾ oz of Whey Protein
10 grams or 0.35 oz of Peanuts

Protein 25g, Fat 7g, Carb 22g, Fibre 8g, 254 Kcals

Preparation

Place the nuts or seeds into the Tall Cup. Screw the Nutribullet Extractor Blade on to the top of the cup. Invert the cup, press it down into the Nutribullet Power Base and twist it into place. Blast them for 30 seconds. Put the rest of the solid ingredients into the cup and press them down below the Max Line. Add the fluid base to fill the cup up to the Max Line. Screw the Nutribullet Extractor Blade on to the top of the cup. Invert the cup, press it down into the Nutribullet Power Base and twist it into place. Blast the mixture until it is really smooth (20 or so seconds). **Enjoy!**

Broccoli and Spinach Tonic

Ingredients

1 Cup/Handful of Broccoli Florets (40 grams or 1½ oz)
1 Cup/Handful of Spinach (40 grams or 1½ oz)
¾ Cup of Blueberries (90 grams or 3 oz)
¾ Cup of Radishes (90 grams or 3 oz)
200 ml / 7 fl oz of Almond Milk (Unsweetened)
25 grams or ¾ oz of Whey Protein
8 grams or 0.28 oz of Pumpkin Seeds

Protein 25g, Fat 8g, Carb 18g, Fibre 9g, 254 Kcals

Preparation

Place the nuts or seeds into the Tall Cup. Screw the Nutribullet Extractor Blade on to the top of the cup. Invert the cup, press it down into the Nutribullet Power Base and twist it into place. Blast them for 30 seconds. Put the rest of the solid ingredients into the cup and press them down below the Max Line. Add the fluid base to fill the cup up to the Max Line. Screw the Nutribullet Extractor Blade on to the top of the cup. Invert the cup, press it down into the Nutribullet Power Base and twist it into place. Blast the mixture until it is really smooth (20 or so seconds). **Enjoy!**

Rocket embraces Grapefruit

Ingredients

1 Cup/Handful of Rocket/Arugura Lettuce (40 grams or 1½ oz)
1 Cup/Handful of Spinach (40 grams or 1½ oz)
¾ Cup of Grapefruit segments (90 grams or 3 oz)
¾ Cup of sliced Celery (90 grams or 3 oz)
200 ml / 7 fl oz of Hazelnut Milk
22 grams or ¾ oz of Soy Protein
8 grams or 0.28 oz of Brazil nuts

Protein 24g, Fat 9g, Carb 16g, Fibre 5g, 254 Kcals

Preparation

Place the nuts or seeds into the Tall Cup. Screw the Nutribullet Extractor Blade on to the top of the cup. Invert the cup, press it down into the Nutribullet Power Base and twist it into place. Blast them for 30 seconds. Put the rest of the solid ingredients into the cup and press them down below the Max Line. Add the fluid base to fill the cup up to the Max Line. Screw the Nutribullet Extractor Blade on to the top of the cup. Invert the cup, press it down into the Nutribullet Power Base and twist it into place. Blast the mixture until it is really smooth (20 or so seconds). **Enjoy!**

Guava befriends Beetroot

Ingredients

1 Cup/Handful of Watercress (40 grams or 1½ oz)
1 Cup/Handful of Lettuce Leaves (40 grams or 1½ oz)
¾ Cup of Guava (90 grams or 3 oz)
¾ Cup of diced Beetroot (90 grams or 3 oz)
200 ml / 7 fl oz of Almond Milk (Unsweetened)
25 grams or ¾ oz of Whey Protein
4 grams or 0.14 oz of Peanuts

Protein 26g, Fat 7g, Carb 17g, Fibre 11g, 254 Kcals

Preparation

Place the nuts or seeds into the Tall Cup. Screw the Nutribullet Extractor Blade on to the top of the cup. Invert the cup, press it down into the Nutribullet Power Base and twist it into place. Blast them for 30 seconds. Put the rest of the solid ingredients into the cup and press them down below the Max Line. Add the fluid base to fill the cup up to the Max Line. Screw the Nutribullet Extractor Blade on to the top of the cup. Invert the cup, press it down into the Nutribullet Power Base and twist it into place. Blast the mixture until it is really smooth (20 or so seconds). **Enjoy!**

Red Pepper Dream

Ingredients

1 Cup/Handful of Green Cabbage (40 grams or 1½ oz)
1 Cup/Handful of Lettuce Leaves (40 grams or 1½ oz)
¾ Cup of Pineapple chunks (90 grams or 3 oz)
¾ Cup of sliced Red Pepper (90 grams or 3 oz)
200 ml / 7 fl oz of Almond Milk (Unsweetened)
25 grams or ¾ oz of Whey Protein
8 grams or 0.28 oz of Cashews

Protein 24g, Fat 7g, Carb 20g, Fibre 8g, 254 Kcals

Preparation

Place the nuts or seeds into the Tall Cup. Screw the Nutribullet Extractor Blade on to the top of the cup. Invert the cup, press it down into the Nutribullet Power Base and twist it into place. Blast them for 30 seconds. Put the rest of the solid ingredients into the cup and press them down below the Max Line. Add the fluid base to fill the cup up to the Max Line. Screw the Nutribullet Extractor Blade on to the top of the cup. Invert the cup, press it down into the Nutribullet Power Base and twist it into place. Blast the mixture until it is really smooth (20 or so seconds). **Enjoy!**

Mint invites Broccoli

Ingredients

1 Cup/Handful of Mint (40 grams or 1½ oz)
1 Cup/Handful of Broccoli Florets (40 grams or 1½ oz)
¾ Cup of Pear slices (90 grams or 3 oz)
¾ Cup of Radishes (90 grams or 3 oz)
200 ml / 7 fl oz of Coconut Milk
25 grams or ¾ oz of Rice Protein
5 grams or 0.18 oz of Chia Seeds

Protein 24g, Fat 4g, Carb 24g, Fibre 10g, 254 Kcals

Preparation

Place the nuts or seeds into the Tall Cup. Screw the Nutribullet Extractor Blade on to the top of the cup. Invert the cup, press it down into the Nutribullet Power Base and twist it into place. Blast them for 30 seconds. Put the rest of the solid ingredients into the cup and press them down below the Max Line. Add the fluid base to fill the cup up to the Max Line. Screw the Nutribullet Extractor Blade on to the top of the cup. Invert the cup, press it down into the Nutribullet Power Base and twist it into place. Blast the mixture until it is really smooth (20 or so seconds). **Enjoy!**

Bok Choy hugs Mango

Ingredients

2 Cups/Handfuls of Bok Choy (80 grams or 3 oz)
¾ Cup of Mango slices (90 grams or 3 oz)
¾ Cup of diced Turnip (90 grams or 3 oz)
200 ml / 7 fl oz of Hazelnut Milk
25 grams or ¾ oz of Pea Protein
1 gram or 0.04 oz of Sunflower Seeds Hulled

Protein 23g, Fat 5g, Carb 26g, Fibre 5g, 254 Kcals

Preparation

Place the nuts or seeds into the Tall Cup. Screw the Nutribullet Extractor Blade on to the top of the cup. Invert the cup, press it down into the Nutribullet Power Base and twist it into place. Blast them for 30 seconds. Put the rest of the solid ingredients into the cup and press them down below the Max Line. Add the fluid base to fill the cup up to the Max Line. Screw the Nutribullet Extractor Blade on to the top of the cup. Invert the cup, press it down into the Nutribullet Power Base and twist it into place. Blast the mixture until it is really smooth (20 or so seconds). **Enjoy!**

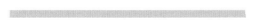

Mint and Peach Vision

Ingredients

1 Cup/Handful of Watercress (40 grams or 1½ oz)
1 Cup/Handful of Mint (40 grams or 1½ oz)
¾ Cup of Peach slices (90 grams or 3 oz)
¾ Cup of diced Swede (90 grams or 3 oz)
200 ml / 7 fl oz of Almond Milk (Unsweetened)
25 grams or ¾ oz of Whey Protein
9 grams or 0.32 oz of Pumpkin Seeds

Protein 26g, Fat 8g, Carb 16g, Fibre 9g, 254 Kcals

Preparation

Place the nuts or seeds into the Tall Cup. Screw the Nutribullet Extractor Blade on to the top of the cup. Invert the cup, press it down into the Nutribullet Power Base and twist it into place. Blast them for 30 seconds. Put the rest of the solid ingredients into the cup and press them down below the Max Line. Add the fluid base to fill the cup up to the Max Line. Screw the Nutribullet Extractor Blade on to the top of the cup. Invert the cup, press it down into the Nutribullet Power Base and twist it into place. Blast the mixture until it is really smooth (20 or so seconds). **Enjoy!**

Grapefruit and Turnip Tango

Ingredients

2 Cups/Handfuls of Mint (80 grams or 3 oz)
¾ Cup of Grapefruit segments (90 grams or 3 oz)
¾ Cup of diced Turnip (90 grams or 3 oz)
200 ml / 7 fl oz of Coconut Milk
25 grams or ¾ oz of Pea Protein
4 grams or 0.14 oz of Almonds

Protein 25g, Fat 5g, Carb 20g, Fibre 8g, 254 Kcals

Preparation

Place the nuts or seeds into the Tall Cup. Screw the Nutribullet Extractor Blade on to the top of the cup. Invert the cup, press it down into the Nutribullet Power Base and twist it into place. Blast them for 30 seconds. Put the rest of the solid ingredients into the cup and press them down below the Max Line. Add the fluid base to fill the cup up to the Max Line. Screw the Nutribullet Extractor Blade on to the top of the cup. Invert the cup, press it down into the Nutribullet Power Base and twist it into place. Blast the mixture until it is really smooth (20 or so seconds). **Enjoy!**

Watercress and Pear Ensemble

Ingredients

1 Cup/Handful of Watercress (40 grams or 1½ oz)
1 Cup/Handful of Broccoli Florets (40 grams or 1½ oz)
¾ Cup of Pear slices (90 grams or 3 oz)
¾ Cup of sliced Red Pepper (90 grams or 3 oz)
200 ml / 7 fl oz of Hazelnut Milk
25 grams or ¾ oz of Whey Protein
1 gram or 0.04 oz of Chia Seeds

Protein 23g, Fat 5g, Carb 25g, Fibre 9g, 254 Kcals

Preparation

Place the nuts or seeds into the Tall Cup. Screw the Nutribullet Extractor Blade on to the top of the cup. Invert the cup, press it down into the Nutribullet Power Base and twist it into place. Blast them for 30 seconds. Put the rest of the solid ingredients into the cup and press them down below the Max Line. Add the fluid base to fill the cup up to the Max Line. Screw the Nutribullet Extractor Blade on to the top of the cup. Invert the cup, press it down into the Nutribullet Power Base and twist it into place. Blast the mixture until it is really smooth (20 or so seconds). **Enjoy!**

Spinach Constellation

Ingredients

1 Cup/Handful of Spinach (40 grams or 1½ oz)
1 Cup/Handful of Bok Choy (40 grams or 1½ oz)
¾ Cup of Blackberries (90 grams or 3 oz)
¾ Cup of sliced Green Pepper (90 grams or 3 oz)
200 ml / 7 fl oz of Coconut Milk
22 grams or ¾ oz of Soy Protein
12 grams or 0.42 oz of Chia Seeds

Protein 26g, Fat 6g, Carb 15g, Fibre 12g, 254 Kcals

Preparation

Place the nuts or seeds into the Tall Cup. Screw the Nutribullet Extractor Blade on to the top of the cup. Invert the cup, press it down into the Nutribullet Power Base and twist it into place. Blast them for 30 seconds. Put the rest of the solid ingredients into the cup and press them down below the Max Line. Add the fluid base to fill the cup up to the Max Line. Screw the Nutribullet Extractor Blade on to the top of the cup. Invert the cup, press it down into the Nutribullet Power Base and twist it into place. Blast the mixture until it is really smooth (20 or so seconds). **Enjoy!**

Orange Explosion

Ingredients

1 Cup/Handful of Spinach (40 grams or 1½ oz)
1 Cup/Handful of Fennel (40 grams or 1½ oz)
¾ Cup of Orange segments (90 grams or 3 oz)
¾ Cup of diced Turnip (90 grams or 3 oz)
200 ml / 7 fl oz of Hazelnut Milk
25 grams or ¾ oz of Pea Protein
1 gram or 0.04 oz of Almonds

Protein 24g, Fat 5g, Carb 24g, Fibre 7g, 254 Kcals

Preparation

Place the nuts or seeds into the Tall Cup. Screw the Nutribullet Extractor Blade on to the top of the cup. Invert the cup, press it down into the Nutribullet Power Base and twist it into place. Blast them for 30 seconds. Put the rest of the solid ingredients into the cup and press them down below the Max Line. Add the fluid base to fill the cup up to the Max Line. Screw the Nutribullet Extractor Blade on to the top of the cup. Invert the cup, press it down into the Nutribullet Power Base and twist it into place. Blast the mixture until it is really smooth (20 or so seconds). **Enjoy!**

Zucchini Reaction

Ingredients

2 Cups/Handfuls of Red or White Cabbage (80 grams or 3 oz)
¾ Cup of Plum halves (90 grams or 3 oz)
¾ Cup of sliced Zucchini/Courgette (90 grams or 3 oz)
200 ml / 7 fl oz of Almond Milk (Unsweetened)
22 grams or ¾ oz of Soy Protein
12 grams or 0.42 oz of Sunflower Seeds Hulled

Protein 26g, Fat 9g, Carb 18g, Fibre 5g, 254 Kcals

Preparation

Place the nuts or seeds into the Tall Cup. Screw the Nutribullet Extractor Blade on to the top of the cup. Invert the cup, press it down into the Nutribullet Power Base and twist it into place. Blast them for 30 seconds. Put the rest of the solid ingredients into the cup and press them down below the Max Line. Add the fluid base to fill the cup up to the Max Line. Screw the Nutribullet Extractor Blade on to the top of the cup. Invert the cup, press it down into the Nutribullet Power Base and twist it into place. Blast the mixture until it is really smooth (20 or so seconds). **Enjoy!**

Fennel embraces Raspberry

Ingredients

1 Cup/Handful of Rocket/Arugura Lettuce (40 grams or 1½ oz)
1 Cup/Handful of Fennel (40 grams or 1½ oz)
¾ Cup of Raspberries (90 grams or 3 oz)
¾ Cup of sliced Cauliflower florets (90 grams or 3 oz)
200 ml / 7 fl oz of Coconut Milk
25 grams or ¾ oz of Rice Protein
6 grams or 0.21 oz of Pumpkin Seeds

Protein 25g, Fat 6g, Carb 18g, Fibre 10g, 254 Kcals

Preparation

Place the nuts or seeds into the Tall Cup. Screw the Nutribullet Extractor Blade on to the top of the cup. Invert the cup, press it down into the Nutribullet Power Base and twist it into place. Blast them for 30 seconds. Put the rest of the solid ingredients into the cup and press them down below the Max Line. Add the fluid base to fill the cup up to the Max Line. Screw the Nutribullet Extractor Blade on to the top of the cup. Invert the cup, press it down into the Nutribullet Power Base and twist it into place. Blast the mixture until it is really smooth (20 or so seconds). **Enjoy!**

Broccoli goes Red Cabbage

Ingredients

1 Cup/Handful of Broccoli Florets (40 grams or 1½ oz)
1 Cup/Handful of Red or White Cabbage (40 grams or 1½ oz)
¾ Cup of Plum halves (90 grams or 3 oz)
¾ Cup of sliced Zucchini/Courgette (90 grams or 3 oz)
200 ml / 7 fl oz of Coconut Milk
25 grams or ¾ oz of Whey Protein
6 grams or 0.21 oz of Hazelnuts

Protein 24g, Fat 7g, Carb 22g, Fibre 6g, 254 Kcals

Preparation

Place the nuts or seeds into the Tall Cup. Screw the Nutribullet Extractor Blade on to the top of the cup. Invert the cup, press it down into the Nutribullet Power Base and twist it into place. Blast them for 30 seconds. Put the rest of the solid ingredients into the cup and press them down below the Max Line. Add the fluid base to fill the cup up to the Max Line. Screw the Nutribullet Extractor Blade on to the top of the cup. Invert the cup, press it down into the Nutribullet Power Base and twist it into place. Blast the mixture until it is really smooth (20 or so seconds). **Enjoy!**

Fig hugs Zucchini

Ingredients

1 Cup/Handful of Bok Choy (40 grams or 1½ oz)
1 Cup/Handful of Lettuce Leaves (40 grams or 1½ oz)
¾ Cup of Peeled Figs (90 grams or 3 oz)
¾ Cup of sliced Zucchini/Courgette (90 grams or 3 oz)
200 ml / 7 fl oz of Water
25 grams or ¾ oz of Pea Protein
9 grams or 0.32 oz of Brazil nuts

Protein 24g, Fat 8g, Carb 21g, Fibre 5g, 254 Kcals

Preparation

Place the nuts or seeds into the Tall Cup. Screw the Nutribullet Extractor Blade on to the top of the cup. Invert the cup, press it down into the Nutribullet Power Base and twist it into place. Blast them for 30 seconds. Put the rest of the solid ingredients into the cup and press them down below the Max Line. Add the fluid base to fill the cup up to the Max Line. Screw the Nutribullet Extractor Blade on to the top of the cup. Invert the cup, press it down into the Nutribullet Power Base and twist it into place. Blast the mixture until it is really smooth (20 or so seconds). **Enjoy!**

Fine Bean Machine

Ingredients

1 Cup/Handful of Watercress (40 grams or 1½ oz)
1 Cup/Handful of Rocket/Arugura Lettuce (40 grams or 1½ oz)
¾ Cup of Cherries (stoned) (90 grams or 3 oz)
¾ Cup of sliced Fine Beans (90 grams or 3 oz)
200 ml / 7 fl oz of Almond Milk (Unsweetened)
25 grams or ¾ oz of Rice Protein
7 grams or 0.25 oz of Brazil nuts

Protein 26g, Fat 8g, Carb 19g, Fibre 6g, 254 Kcals

Preparation

Place the nuts or seeds into the Tall Cup. Screw the Nutribullet Extractor Blade on to the top of the cup. Invert the cup, press it down into the Nutribullet Power Base and twist it into place. Blast them for 30 seconds. Put the rest of the solid ingredients into the cup and press them down below the Max Line. Add the fluid base to fill the cup up to the Max Line. Screw the Nutribullet Extractor Blade on to the top of the cup. Invert the cup, press it down into the Nutribullet Power Base and twist it into place. Blast the mixture until it is really smooth (20 or so seconds). **Enjoy!**

Fennel and Plum Energizer

Ingredients

1 Cup/Handful of Fennel (40 grams or 1½ oz)
1 Cup/Handful of Green Cabbage (40 grams or 1½ oz)
¾ Cup of Plum halves (90 grams or 3 oz)
¾ Cup of sliced Green Pepper (90 grams or 3 oz)
200 ml / 7 fl oz of Hazelnut Milk
25 grams or ¾ oz of Whey Protein
3 grams or 0.11 oz of Pecans

Protein 22g, Fat 7g, Carb 23g, Fibre 8g, 255 Kcals

Preparation

Place the nuts or seeds into the Tall Cup. Screw the Nutribullet Extractor Blade on to the top of the cup. Invert the cup, press it down into the Nutribullet Power Base and twist it into place. Blast them for 30 seconds. Put the rest of the solid ingredients into the cup and press them down below the Max Line. Add the fluid base to fill the cup up to the Max Line. Screw the Nutribullet Extractor Blade on to the top of the cup. Invert the cup, press it down into the Nutribullet Power Base and twist it into place. Blast the mixture until it is really smooth (20 or so seconds). **Enjoy!**

Apple and Tomato Melody

Ingredients

1 Cup/Handful of Spinach (40 grams or 1½ oz)
1 Cup/Handful of Watercress (40 grams or 1½ oz)
¾ Cup of Apple slices (90 grams or 3 oz)
¾ Cup of sliced Tomato (90 grams or 3 oz)
200 ml / 7 fl oz of Almond Milk (Unsweetened)
22 grams or ¾ oz of Soy Protein
13 grams or 0.46 oz of Sunflower Seeds Hulled

Protein 26g, Fat 9g, Carb 17g, Fibre 6g, 255 Kcals

Preparation

Place the nuts or seeds into the Tall Cup. Screw the Nutribullet Extractor Blade on to the top of the cup. Invert the cup, press it down into the Nutribullet Power Base and twist it into place. Blast them for 30 seconds. Put the rest of the solid ingredients into the cup and press them down below the Max Line. Add the fluid base to fill the cup up to the Max Line. Screw the Nutribullet Extractor Blade on to the top of the cup. Invert the cup, press it down into the Nutribullet Power Base and twist it into place. Blast the mixture until it is really smooth (20 or so seconds). **Enjoy!**

Apple and Yellow Pepper Surprise

Ingredients

1 Cup/Handful of Spinach (40 grams or 1½ oz)
1 Cup/Handful of Watercress (40 grams or 1½ oz)
¾ Cup of Apple slices (90 grams or 3 oz)
¾ Cup of sliced Yellow Pepper (90 grams or 3 oz)
200 ml / 7 fl oz of Almond Milk (Unsweetened)
25 grams or ¾ oz of Pea Protein
8 grams or 0.28 oz of Flax Seeds

Protein 25g, Fat 7g, Carb 18g, Fibre 7g, 255 Kcals

Preparation

Place the nuts or seeds into the Tall Cup. Screw the Nutribullet Extractor Blade on to the top of the cup. Invert the cup, press it down into the Nutribullet Power Base and twist it into place. Blast them for 30 seconds. Put the rest of the solid ingredients into the cup and press them down below the Max Line. Add the fluid base to fill the cup up to the Max Line. Screw the Nutribullet Extractor Blade on to the top of the cup. Invert the cup, press it down into the Nutribullet Power Base and twist it into place. Blast the mixture until it is really smooth (20 or so seconds). *Enjoy!*

Lettuce befriends Apple

Ingredients

1 Cup/Handful of Broccoli Florets (40 grams or 1½ oz)
1 Cup/Handful of Lettuce Leaves (40 grams or 1½ oz)
¾ Cup of Apple slices (90 grams or 3 oz)
¾ Cup of sliced Fine Beans (90 grams or 3 oz)
200 ml / 7 fl oz of Coconut Milk
25 grams or ¾ oz of Pea Protein
4 grams or 0.14 oz of Sesame Seeds Hulled

Protein 24g, Fat 6g, Carb 23g, Fibre 6g, 255 Kcals

Preparation

Place the nuts or seeds into the Tall Cup. Screw the Nutribullet Extractor Blade on to the top of the cup. Invert the cup, press it down into the Nutribullet Power Base and twist it into place. Blast them for 30 seconds. Put the rest of the solid ingredients into the cup and press them down below the Max Line. Add the fluid base to fill the cup up to the Max Line. Screw the Nutribullet Extractor Blade on to the top of the cup. Invert the cup, press it down into the Nutribullet Power Base and twist it into place. Blast the mixture until it is really smooth (20 or so seconds). *Enjoy!*

Lettuce and Mango City

Ingredients

1 Cup/Handful of Green Cabbage (40 grams or 1½ oz)
1 Cup/Handful of Lettuce Leaves (40 grams or 1½ oz)
¾ Cup of Mango slices (90 grams or 3 oz)
¾ Cup of sliced Zucchini/Courgette (90 grams or 3 oz)
200 ml / 7 fl oz of Hazelnut Milk
22 grams or ¾ oz of Soy Protein
4 grams or 0.14 oz of Walnuts

Protein 24g, Fat 7g, Carb 23g, Fibre 5g, 255 Kcals

Preparation

Place the nuts or seeds into the Tall Cup. Screw the Nutribullet Extractor Blade on to the top of the cup. Invert the cup, press it down into the Nutribullet Power Base and twist it into place. Blast them for 30 seconds. Put the rest of the solid ingredients into the cup and press them down below the Max Line. Add the fluid base to fill the cup up to the Max Line. Screw the Nutribullet Extractor Blade on to the top of the cup. Invert the cup, press it down into the Nutribullet Power Base and twist it into place. Blast the mixture until it is really smooth (20 or so seconds). **Enjoy!**

Rocket goes Fennel

Ingredients

1 Cup/Handful of Rocket/Arugura Lettuce (40 grams or 1½ oz)
1 Cup/Handful of Fennel (40 grams or 1½ oz)
¾ Cup of Blackberries (90 grams or 3 oz)
¾ Cup of sliced Cucumber (90 grams or 3 oz)
200 ml / 7 fl oz of Coconut Milk
22 grams or ¾ oz of Soy Protein
11 grams or 0.39 oz of Peanuts

Protein 26g, Fat 8g, Carb 15g, Fibre 8g, 255 Kcals

Preparation

Place the nuts or seeds into the Tall Cup. Screw the Nutribullet Extractor Blade on to the top of the cup. Invert the cup, press it down into the Nutribullet Power Base and twist it into place. Blast them for 30 seconds. Put the rest of the solid ingredients into the cup and press them down below the Max Line. Add the fluid base to fill the cup up to the Max Line. Screw the Nutribullet Extractor Blade on to the top of the cup. Invert the cup, press it down into the Nutribullet Power Base and twist it into place. Blast the mixture until it is really smooth (20 or so seconds). **Enjoy!**

Clementine Regatta

Ingredients

1 Cup/Handful of Fennel (40 grams or 1½ oz)
1 Cup/Handful of Red or White Cabbage (40 grams or 1½ oz)
¾ Cup of Clementine slices (90 grams or 3 oz)
¾ Cup of sliced Celery (90 grams or 3 oz)
200 ml / 7 fl oz of Hazelnut Milk
25 grams or ¾ oz of Rice Protein
4 grams or 0.14 oz of Peanuts

Protein 24g, Fat 6g, Carb 23g, Fibre 6g, 255 Kcals

Preparation

Place the nuts or seeds into the Tall Cup. Screw the Nutribullet Extractor Blade on to the top of the cup. Invert the cup, press it down into the Nutribullet Power Base and twist it into place. Blast them for 30 seconds. Put the rest of the solid ingredients into the cup and press them down below the Max Line. Add the fluid base to fill the cup up to the Max Line. Screw the Nutribullet Extractor Blade on to the top of the cup. Invert the cup, press it down into the Nutribullet Power Base and twist it into place. Blast the mixture until it is really smooth (20 or so seconds). **Enjoy!**

Lettuce Perfection

Ingredients

1 Cup/Handful of Bok Choy (40 grams or 1½ oz)
1 Cup/Handful of Lettuce Leaves (40 grams or 1½ oz)
¾ Cup of Papaya (90 grams or 3 oz)
¾ Cup of sliced Green Pepper (90 grams or 3 oz)
200 ml / 7 fl oz of Water
25 grams or ¾ oz of Whey Protein
14 grams or 0.49 oz of Brazil nuts

Protein 23g, Fat 11g, Carb 14g, Fibre 7g, 255 Kcals

Preparation

Place the nuts or seeds into the Tall Cup. Screw the Nutribullet Extractor Blade on to the top of the cup. Invert the cup, press it down into the Nutribullet Power Base and twist it into place. Blast them for 30 seconds. Put the rest of the solid ingredients into the cup and press them down below the Max Line. Add the fluid base to fill the cup up to the Max Line. Screw the Nutribullet Extractor Blade on to the top of the cup. Invert the cup, press it down into the Nutribullet Power Base and twist it into place. Blast the mixture until it is really smooth (20 or so seconds). **Enjoy!**

Rocket joins Mint

Ingredients

1 Cup/Handful of Rocket/Arugura Lettuce (40 grams or 1½ oz)
1 Cup/Handful of Mint (40 grams or 1½ oz)
¾ Cup of Melon chunks (90 grams or 3 oz)
¾ Cup of sliced Zucchini/Courgette (90 grams or 3 oz)
200 ml / 7 fl oz of Hazelnut Milk
22 grams or ¾ oz of Soy Protein
7 grams or 0.25 oz of Almonds

Protein 25g, Fat 8g, Carb 18g, Fibre 6g, 255 Kcals

Preparation

Place the nuts or seeds into the Tall Cup. Screw the Nutribullet Extractor Blade on to the top of the cup. Invert the cup, press it down into the Nutribullet Power Base and twist it into place. Blast them for 30 seconds. Put the rest of the solid ingredients into the cup and press them down below the Max Line. Add the fluid base to fill the cup up to the Max Line. Screw the Nutribullet Extractor Blade on to the top of the cup. Invert the cup, press it down into the Nutribullet Power Base and twist it into place. Blast the mixture until it is really smooth (20 or so seconds). **Enjoy!**

Broccoli and Fig Morning

Ingredients

1 Cup/Handful of Lettuce Leaves (40 grams or 1½ oz)
1 Cup/Handful of Broccoli Florets (40 grams or 1½ oz)
¾ Cup of Peeled Figs (90 grams or 3 oz)
¾ Cup of diced Turnip (90 grams or 3 oz)
200 ml / 7 fl oz of Water
25 grams or ¾ oz of Pea Protein
7 grams or 0.25 oz of Sesame Seeds Hulled

Protein 24g, Fat 5g, Carb 24g, Fibre 7g, 255 Kcals

Preparation

Place the nuts or seeds into the Tall Cup. Screw the Nutribullet Extractor Blade on to the top of the cup. Invert the cup, press it down into the Nutribullet Power Base and twist it into place. Blast them for 30 seconds. Put the rest of the solid ingredients into the cup and press them down below the Max Line. Add the fluid base to fill the cup up to the Max Line. Screw the Nutribullet Extractor Blade on to the top of the cup. Invert the cup, press it down into the Nutribullet Power Base and twist it into place. Blast the mixture until it is really smooth (20 or so seconds). **Enjoy!**

Blackberry Supermodel

Ingredients

1 Cup/Handful of Spinach (40 grams or 1½ oz)
1 Cup/Handful of Mint (40 grams or 1½ oz)
¾ Cup of Blackberries (90 grams or 3 oz)
¾ Cup of sliced Zucchini/Courgette (90 grams or 3 oz)
200 ml / 7 fl oz of Coconut Milk
25 grams or ¾ oz of Rice Protein
7 grams or 0.25 oz of Sesame Seeds Hulled

Protein 26g, Fat 7g, Carb 15g, Fibre 10g, 255 Kcals

Preparation

Place the nuts or seeds into the Tall Cup. Screw the Nutribullet Extractor Blade on to the top of the cup. Invert the cup, press it down into the Nutribullet Power Base and twist it into place. Blast them for 30 seconds. Put the rest of the solid ingredients into the cup and press them down below the Max Line. Add the fluid base to fill the cup up to the Max Line. Screw the Nutribullet Extractor Blade on to the top of the cup. Invert the cup, press it down into the Nutribullet Power Base and twist it into place. Blast the mixture until it is really smooth (20 or so seconds). *Enjoy!*

Kiwi and Carrot Snog

Ingredients

1 Cup/Handful of Bok Choy (40 grams or 1½ oz)
1 Cup/Handful of Lettuce Leaves (40 grams or 1½ oz)
¾ Cup of Kiwi Fruit slices (90 grams or 3 oz)
¾ Cup of sliced Carrots (90 grams or 3 oz)
200 ml / 7 fl oz of Water
25 grams or ¾ oz of Rice Protein
9 grams or 0.32 oz of Walnuts

Protein 24g, Fat 7g, Carb 21g, Fibre 7g, 255 Kcals

Preparation

Place the nuts or seeds into the Tall Cup. Screw the Nutribullet Extractor Blade on to the top of the cup. Invert the cup, press it down into the Nutribullet Power Base and twist it into place. Blast them for 30 seconds. Put the rest of the solid ingredients into the cup and press them down below the Max Line. Add the fluid base to fill the cup up to the Max Line. Screw the Nutribullet Extractor Blade on to the top of the cup. Invert the cup, press it down into the Nutribullet Power Base and twist it into place. Blast the mixture until it is really smooth (20 or so seconds). *Enjoy!*

Cranberry Chorus

Ingredients

2 Cups/Handfuls of Spinach (80 grams or 3 oz)
¾ Cup of Cranberries (90 grams or 3 oz)
¾ Cup of sliced Tomato (90 grams or 3 oz)
200 ml / 7 fl oz of Hazelnut Milk
25 grams or ¾ oz of Whey Protein
4 grams or 0.14 oz of Pecans

Protein 23g, Fat 8g, Carb 19g, Fibre 10g, 256 Kcals

Preparation

Place the nuts or seeds into the Tall Cup. Screw the Nutribullet Extractor Blade on to the top of the cup. Invert the cup, press it down into the Nutribullet Power Base and twist it into place. Blast them for 30 seconds. Put the rest of the solid ingredients into the cup and press them down below the Max Line. Add the fluid base to fill the cup up to the Max Line. Screw the Nutribullet Extractor Blade on to the top of the cup. Invert the cup, press it down into the Nutribullet Power Base and twist it into place. Blast the mixture until it is really smooth (20 or so seconds). **Enjoy!**

Apricot Concerto

Ingredients

2 Cups/Handfuls of Watercress (80 grams or 3 oz)
¾ Cup of Apricot halves (90 grams or 3 oz)
¾ Cup of diced Turnip (90 grams or 3 oz)
200 ml / 7 fl oz of Coconut Milk
25 grams or ¾ oz of Rice Protein
7 grams or 0.25 oz of Walnuts

Protein 25g, Fat 7g, Carb 21g, Fibre 4g, 256 Kcals

Preparation

Place the nuts or seeds into the Tall Cup. Screw the Nutribullet Extractor Blade on to the top of the cup. Invert the cup, press it down into the Nutribullet Power Base and twist it into place. Blast them for 30 seconds. Put the rest of the solid ingredients into the cup and press them down below the Max Line. Add the fluid base to fill the cup up to the Max Line. Screw the Nutribullet Extractor Blade on to the top of the cup. Invert the cup, press it down into the Nutribullet Power Base and twist it into place. Blast the mixture until it is really smooth (20 or so seconds). **Enjoy!**

NOTES

NOTES

NOTES

Printed in Great Britain
by Amazon.co.uk, Ltd.,
Marston Gate.